INTEGRATING HOLISTIC WELLNESS AND ENVIRONMENTAL SUSTAINABILITY

A COMPREHENSIVE APPROACH TO MODERN HEALTH CHALLENGES

DR. RALPH LEEBEN J

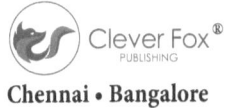

Chennai • Bangalore

CLEVER FOX PUBLISHING
Chennai, India

Published by CLEVER FOX PUBLISHING 2024
Copyright © Dr.Ralph Leeben J 2024

All Rights Reserved.
ISBN: 978-93-67078-62-4

This book has been published with all reasonable efforts taken to make the material error-free after the consent of the author. No part of this book shall be used, reproduced in any manner whatsoever without written permission from the author, except in the case of brief quotations embodied in critical articles and reviews.

The Author of this book is solely responsible and liable for its content including but not limited to the views, representations, descriptions, statements, information, opinions and references ["Content"]. The Content of this book shall not constitute or be construed or deemed to reflect the opinion or expression of the Publisher or Editor. Neither the Publisher nor Editor endorse or approve the Content of this book or guarantee the reliability, accuracy or completeness of the Content published herein and do not make any representations or warranties of any kind, express or implied, including but not limited to the implied warranties of merchantability, fitness for a particular purpose. The Publisher and Editor shall not be liable whatsoever for any errors, omissions, whether such errors or omissions result from negligence, accident, or any other cause or claims for loss or damages of any kind, including without limitation, indirect or consequential loss or damage arising out of use, inability to use, or about the reliability, accuracy or sufficiency of the information contained in this book.

In Loving Memory of My Father

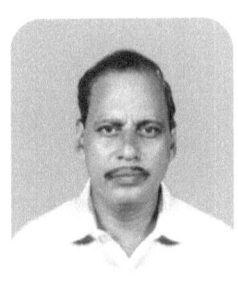

(Late)Mr. A. Jacob Bensam, M.A., M.Ed.

Retired Teacher

"A distinguished source of inspiration."

CONTENTS

Foreword .... *vii*
Prolog .... *ix*
Recommendation .... *xi*
About Author .... *xiii*

1. Introduction 1
2. Harmful Chemicals in Everyday Products 3
3. Toxic-Free Taste 28
4. Digital Dilemmas 37
5. Behavioral and Character Changes and Excessive Electronic Gadget Use 45
6. Mindful Eating 50
7. The Effects of Pesticides on Ecosystems and People 53
8. Managing Exposure to Food Additives and Preservatives 78
9. A Review on Food Adulteration 91
10. The Health and Dental Implications of Carbonated Beverages 109
11. Strategies for Pollution Control and Human Health Protection 115
12. Challenges and Strategies in Ensuring Safe Drinking Water 128
13. Health Benefits With Antioxidants and Nutritional Supplements 140
14. Optimal Health Through Nutrient-Rich Foods 159

Contents

15. Guide to Avoid Harmful Food Combinations 166
16. Nutritional Profile of Exotic Fruits 176
17. Nature's Medicine for a Healthy Lifestyle 206
18. Exploring the Healing Power of Herbs 241
19. Balancing Mineral Intake 295
20. The Multidimensional Benefits of Natural Honey and its Derivatives 306
21. Optimizing Your Fitness Routine 315
22. Spectrum of Alternative Therapies 324

References: *345*

FOREWORD

*I*n a world marked by increasing health risks and environmental challenges, "Integrating Holistic Wellness and Environmental Sustainability" serves as a vital resource for those striving to enhance their well-being while making sustainable choices. This comprehensive guide empowers readers to make informed decisions that foster both personal health and planetary stewardship.

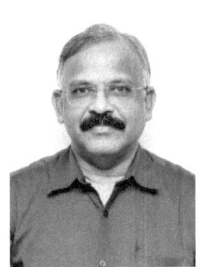

With a strong foundation in practical insights and scientific research, this document explores the invisible threats in our daily lives, such as harmful chemicals in household items, food additives, and cookware materials. Through heightened awareness of these risks, readers are equipped to select safer, non-toxic products and adopt healthier habits that minimize their exposure to potential hazards.

A unique feature of this guide is its emphasis on balanced nutrition, featuring insights into the benefits of superfoods, antioxidants, and essential minerals. It promotes a diet that not only supports physical health but also boosts immune function, energy levels, and longevity. By understanding the health impacts of certain foods and toxic-free cooking practices, readers can take proactive steps toward improved wellness.

Foreword

In addition, this document addresses the mental and emotional toll of modern lifestyles. Sections on digital health caution against the overuse of electronic gadgets, which can lead to stress, anxiety, and reduced attention span. With strategies for mindful digital consumption, readers can foster better mental clarity and emotional resilience.

This work further delves into holistic wellness, exploring the healing potential of natural remedies, herbal therapies, and alternative medicine. By presenting a spectrum of options from acupuncture to herbal treatments, it encourages a multidimensional approach to health that encompasses mind, body, and spirit.

Ultimately, "Integrating Holistic Wellness and Environmental Sustainability" is more than a guide—it is an invitation to a lifestyle that prioritizes wellness and environmental responsibility. Through informed consumer choices, sustainable practices, and preventive health measures, readers can cultivate a balanced, resilient life. May this document inspire meaningful change that enhances individual health and contributes to a healthier, more sustainable world.

Yours Cordially

Dr. R. Anbu Rajan
B.Sc., MBBS, DMLS, FHM, DFM, FCGP
Peace Health Centre, Tirunelveli

PROLOG

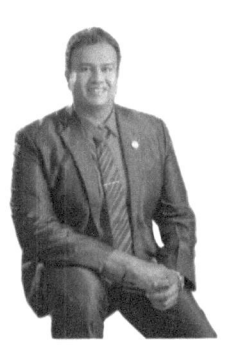

*W*elcome to this interesting green and sustainable "alternative medicine" healthcare approach, I am Dr Prakash an Orthopedic Surgeon and also a qualified alternative medicine practitioner. I am totally amazed as the founder of this book Dr.J. Ralph Leeben have indeed gone beyond in doing an in-depth study of it's the fusion with environment, waste management pollution controls and its compliances (air, water, soil degradation, chemical, toxicity). Infact, beyond this he has also spelled out the spectrum of staying healthy with proper usage of super foods, herbs, honey, and vegetables inline to maximizing of the needful antioxidant and nutritional supplements to stay healthy together with the right healing processes which includes knowledge and fitness therapies.

With our rapid evolving world, high usage of electronic gadgets is unavoidable thus we are exposed to various sort of radiation where the risks are abundance along with our daily cooking wares and pesticide usage coupled with food adulteration. All these are addressed completely in this text with in depth studies and qualified references.

My take, in conclusion is that surpassing the alternative medicine approach, we need to dig deep into the various green practices that can be implemented within the industry to reduce its carbon footprint, minimize waste generation, and prioritize environmental stewardship. From all the medical entities to research institutions and pharmaceutical companies, sustainability initiatives are gaining momentum, making it possible to provide quality healthcare while nurturing the health of mankind. Thus a continuous exploration, of innovative ways, addressing the challenges of climate and environmental degradation is a must adhered formula today to prevail in this industry.

I would like to congratulate Dr, Ralph Leeben ....who have provided successfully the above mentioned solutions, sharing a lot insights of the industry and have delved into the potential benefits that are sustainable to healthcare practices bringing to both patients and the environment. Not forgetting his team and the stakeholders' collaboration, and the ethical implications of sustainable healthcare.

Thank you and shall trust in God to guide you further in your endurance.

Your's sincerely

Dr. Prakash
MBBS, MS (Ortho), MD (Alt. Med)
KL Malysia

RECOMMENDATION

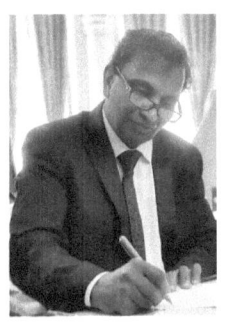

In today's rapidly changing world, addressing health challenges through environmentally friendly approaches has become increasingly vital. The pervasive issue of environmental pollution, coupled with the indiscriminate use of electronic devices, has led to significant physiological and psychological changes in the younger generation. This book serves as a motivational resource, encouraging readers to adopt Holistic Wellness programs that promote a healthier lifestyle.

The book is structured into 22 informative chapters, each dedicated to exploring the hazards associated with harmful chemicals commonly found in everyday products. It provides comprehensive guidance on how individuals can improve their quality of life by ensuring food safety, accessing clean drinking water, and adopting eco-friendly practices. These changes not only contribute to a healthier lifestyle but also promise to reduce unnecessary medical expenses over time.

Additionally, the text emphasizes the critical importance of maintaining a balanced diet and the role of antioxidants in achieving optimal health and fitness. Dr. J. Ralph Leeben, an engineer who earned his PhD from Anna University, has a longstanding passion for environmental conservation. His commitment to this cause has inspired him to write this book, aiming to raise awareness among the public, particularly the youth of the 21st century, about the dangers posed by chemical-based products.

By engaging with this book and actively practicing the suggestions it offers, readers can embark on a transformative journey toward a healthier life. I sincerely wish all readers success in their pursuit of health and well-being.

Dr. J. Ebanasar Msc ,PhD
Principal
Govt Arts & Science College, Modakkurachi, Erode (DT)

ABOUT AUTHOR

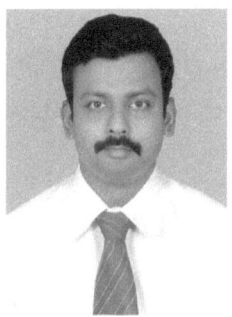

$\mathcal{D}$r. Ralph Leeben is a distinguished expert whose diverse educational background and holistic approach to wellness have made a significant impact on health awareness. After earning his doctorate in Supply Chain Management, Dr. Leeben pursued a path dedicated to holistic health and well-being. He obtained a Master Diploma in Diet & Nutrition, equipping him with comprehensive knowledge of dietary strategies for optimal health.

In his quest to integrate traditional healing techniques with modern wellness practices, Dr. Leeben underwent rigorous training in Bone Setting using the Kalari method, an ancient martial art from Kerala, India, renowned for its therapeutic efficacy. Further enhancing his expertise, he completed a Diploma in Ayurvedic & Panchakarma Therapy, which deepened his understanding of natural healing processes and holistic health management.

Driven by a passion for addressing modern health challenges, Dr. Leeben authored the book **"Integrating Holistic Wellness**

and Environmental Sustainability." In this work, he explores the intricate connection between personal health and the environment, offering practical solutions and insights for managing health in today's fast-paced world. His book serves as a guide for those seeking a balanced approach to health, emphasizing the importance of sustainability and integrated wellness practices. Through his work, Dr. Leeben aims to inspire individuals to lead healthier, more sustainable lives.

1

INTRODUCTION

*N*owadays, with everything going at a million miles per hour, of life seem never-ending, and the environment is rife with health risks, the value of taking a comprehensive view of health cannot be overstated. "Integrating Holistic Wellness and Environmental Sustainability " is not just a book; it's a comprehensive guide that seeks to provide people with the knowledge and resources they need to lead healthier, more balanced lives in the face of today's health challenges.

This guide delves deep into the intricate web of health, shedding light on various aspects that impact our well-being. Starting with the harmful impacts of pollution on people's health and moving on to the hidden dangers posed by food adulteration, pesticides, and even everyday cookware, this book leaves no stone unturned. It emphasizes the significance of fueling our bodies with nutritious foods, engaging in regular physical activity, and embracing the healing powers of nature therapy and treatments.

By delving into the latest research findings and providing practical advice, " Integrating Holistic Wellness and Environmental Sustainability " acts as a guiding light for those navigating the

About Author

maze of modern health challenges. Whether you're on a quest to detoxify your body, strengthen your immune system, or simply savor the natural goodness of honey and herbs, this guide offers a treasure trove of information to encourage you as you strive for a better, more energetic lifestyle.

Come explore with us the hidden relationship between nature and wellness on this illuminating adventure. Find out the best approach embracing a holistic lifestyle can work wonders in transforming your well-being from the inside out. Let's embark on this transformative path together and witness the magic that unfolds when we align ourselves with the healing powers of nature and prioritize holistic wellness in our lives.

2

HARMFUL CHEMICALS IN EVERYDAY PRODUCTS

*I*n our modern world, everyday materials and products often contain hidden chemicals that pose significant health and environmental risks. Here we explore the pervasive presence of these substances in common household items, from furniture and textiles to food packaging and personal care products. By examining the potential hazards associated with chemicals like bisphenol A (BPA), phthalates, formaldehyde, and volatile organic compounds (VOCs), we aim to raise awareness and provide actionable strategies for minimizing exposure. As consumers become more informed, they can make safer choices, advocate for healthier alternatives, and support sustainable practices that ensure the safety of both people and the planet.

Water Bottles and Food Containers

1. BPA, or bisphenol A:

Properties and Use: Polycarbonate plastics and epoxy resins contain the chemical component bisphenol A (BPA). It's a typical component of rigid plastics like water bottles and food containers.

Health Concerns: BPA is known to be it has the potential to alter the body's hormonal systems, making it an endocrine disruptor. It mimics estrogen, a hormone that regulates many biological processes.

Associated Health Risks: Exposure to BPA has a history of association with a number of diseases and conditions, including obesity, cardiovascular disease, and malignancies (including prostate and breast cancer). It can also affect brain development and behavior in fetuses and young children.

2. Phthalates:

Properties and Use: Plastics are made more malleable and less easily broken by adding phthalates, a class of chemicals. Food containers are a common place to find them, plastic wraps, and even in some water bottles.

Health Concerns: Similar to BPA, phthalates are also endocrine disruptors. They can interfere with hormonal balance and have been shown to affect reproductive health.

Associated Health Risks: In children, exposure to phthalates can lead to developmental issues, such as reduced fertility and altered reproductive development. There is also concern about their potential role in conditions like asthma and allergies.

Vinyl Flooring and Plastic Packaging

1. Phthalates and Plasticizers:

Properties and Use: Vinyl flooring and plastic packaging often contain phthalates and other plasticizers to enhance flexibility. These chemicals can off-gas or leach into the environment.

Exposure Risks: Inhalation of these chemicals is a common exposure route, especially in indoor environments where ventilation may be limited. Contact with food can also lead to ingestion.

Associated Health Risks: Prolonged exposure to phthalates and plasticizers can contribute to hormonal imbalances, potentially leading to issues like thyroid dysfunction and reproductive health problems. In children, there is a risk of developmental delays and behavioral issues.

Personal care items such as shampoos, lotions, cosmetics, deodorants, and antiperspirants are commonly used in daily routines. However, they can contain certain chemicals that raise health concerns:

Shampoos, Lotions, and Cosmetics:

1. Parabens:

Function: Parabens are utilized as cosmetic and personal care product preservatives to inhibit the formation of mold and bacteria, therefore prolonging the items' shelf life.

Health Concerns: Parabens have been found in human breast tumors, which has raised concerns about their potential role in cancer development. They are suspected of being endocrine disruptors, meaning it's possible for them to mess with your hormones. There is a chance that this interference might cause problems with reproduction developmental disorders, and an increased risk of certain cancers.

2. Triclosan:

Function: Triclosan is an antibacterial and antifungal agent added to many consumer products, including toothpaste, soaps, and deodorants, to reduce or prevent bacterial contamination.

Health Concerns: Triclosan is thought to disrupt hormones in the body, particularly thyroid hormones, which can affect metabolism and growth. It has also been connected to an elevated danger of some cancers. Additionally, there are concerns about its contribution to antibiotic resistance.

3. Phthalates:

Function: Phthalates are used to make plastics more flexible and are also found in many personal care products such as shampoos and lotions to help dissolve other ingredients.

Health Concerns: Like parabens, phthalates are considered endocrine disruptors. They have been linked to reproductive and developmental issues, particularly in males, and may also be associated with asthma, obesity, and other health concerns.

Deodorants and Antiperspirants:
1. Aluminum Compounds:

Function: Aluminum compounds are used in antiperspirants to temporarily block sweat ducts and reduce perspiration.

Health Concerns: There are concerns that aluminum exposure may be linked to neurological disorders, including Alzheimer's disease. However, the evidence is not conclusive, and more research is needed to determine the extent of these potential risks.

2. Parabens:

Function: As with other personal care products, parabens are used in deodorants and antiperspirants as preservatives.

Health Concerns: The potential endocrine-disrupting effects of parabens in these products can lead to hormone imbalances and associated health risks, similar to those mentioned for shampoos and lotions.

Given these concerns, there is growing interest in natural and organic personal care products that avoid these chemicals. Consumers are advised to read product labels carefully and consider alternatives that are free of these potentially harmful ingredients.

All-Purpose Cleaners and Disinfectants:
1. Chemicals that Emit Volatile Organic Compounds:

Function: Vaporous organic compounds (VOCs) are a class of used in many household products, including cleaning agents, for their solvent properties.

Health and Environmental Concerns: VOCs may dissipate into thin air, adding to the problem of polluting the air inside buildings. Respiratory problems, eye discomfort, headaches, and vertigo may result from prolonged exposure to volatile organic compounds (VOCs). Serious health complications, including as damage to the liver, kidneys, and central nervous system, might develop with prolonged exposure. To further worsen air quality, VOCs help create smog and ground-level ozone.

2. Ammonia:

Function: Since ammonia is so good at removing oil and dirt, it is included in many cleaning products.

Health Concerns: Inhaling ammonia fumes may induce respiratory discomfort and irritate the eyes, nose, and throat. Individuals with asthma or other respiratory conditions may be particularly sensitive to ammonia fumes.

3. Chlorine:

Function: Chlorine is used as a disinfectant to kill bacteria and viruses in water and on surfaces.

Health and Environmental Concerns: Chlorine can react with organic materials to produce harmful byproducts like dioxins, which are contaminants with a long half-life that end up in our food supply. Chlorine exposure can also cause skin and eye irritation, and inhalation of chlorine fumes can lead to respiratory issues.

Laundry Detergents and Fabric Softeners:

1. Fragrances:

Function: Fragrances are added to laundry products to provide a pleasant scent.

Health Concerns: Synthetic fragrances can cause allergic reactions, skin irritation, and respiratory issues in sensitive individuals. They may also contain phthalates, which are endocrine disruptors.

2. Dyes:

Function: Dyes are used to give laundry products a distinctive color.

Health Concerns: Some synthetic dyes can cause skin irritation and allergic reactions. Additionally, they can contribute to water pollution when washed down the drain.

3. Alkyl phenol Ethoxylates (APEs):

Function: APEs are used as surfactants in some detergents and fabric softeners to help remove stains and soften fabrics.

Health and Environmental Concerns: APEs are known to be endocrine disruptors, interfering with hormone function. They are particularly toxic to aquatic life, and their persistence in the environment can lead to long-term ecological harm.

Health Risks Associated with Bisphenol A (BPA) Exposure

Bisphenol A (BPA) is a synthetic chemical used in the production of polycarbonate plastics and epoxy resins, which are found in various consumer products, including thermal paper products like receipts. BPA can leach out of these materials and be absorbed through the skin or ingested, leading to several potential health risks:

1. **Endocrine Disruption**: BPA can mimic estrogen, an essential hormone for human health. Hormonal abnormalities may

result from this disturbance, affecting functions such as growth, development, and reproduction.
2. **Reproductive and Developmental Issues**: BPA exposure has been linked to fertility problems and developmental abnormalities. It may disrupt the proper maturation of a developing baby's brain and reproductive systems.
3. **Heart Health**: Research indicates that exposure to BPA may impact blood pressure and heart function, which in turn may raise the risk of hypertension and heart disease.
4. **Cancer Risk**: There is concern that BPA exposure might increase the estrogen-like effects that increase the risk of malignancies including prostate and breast cancer.
5. **Metabolic Effects**: BPA has been implicated in metabolic disorders, including obesity and insulin resistance, which could contribute to diabetes.
6. **Neurobehavioral Problems**: In children, BPA exposure has been associated with behavioral issues, such as hyperactivity and difficulties with learning and attention.
7. **General Toxicity**: Some studies have shown that BPA can have broader toxicological effects, potentially impacting the liver, kidneys, and overall immune system function

Particleboard and Plywood:
1. Formaldehyde:

Function: Formaldehyde is used in the adhesives and resins that bind wood particles or veneers together in particleboard and plywood. It is prized for its strong bonding properties and cost-effectiveness.

Health Concerns: Formaldehyde is a volatile organic compound (VOC) and a known carcinogen. Exposure to formaldehyde can occur through inhalation of its fumes, which can lead to a range of health issues, including:

Respiratory problems: Coughing, wheezing, and shortness of breath, particularly in individuals with asthma or other respiratory conditions.

Skin irritation: Contact with formaldehyde can cause rashes and other skin reactions.

Eye, nose, and throat irritation: Short-term exposure can result in burning sensations in these areas.

Long-term exposure: Linked to an increased risk of certain types of cancer, particularly nasopharyngeal cancer and leukemia.

Paints and Varnishes:
1. VOCs, or volatile organic compounds:
Function: VOCs are chemical compounds that are used in paints and varnishes to improve application properties, such as drying time and finish quality.

Health and Environmental Concerns: When paint or varnish is applied, VOCs are released into the air as the product dries, contributing to indoor air pollution. Exposure to VOCs can result in:

Eye, nose, and throat irritation: Short-term exposure can lead to discomfort and irritation in these areas.

Headaches, dizziness, and nausea: Inhalation of VOCs can affect the central nervous system and lead to these symptoms.

Poor indoor air quality: VOCs contribute to the formation of smog and ground-level ozone, exacerbating air pollution issues indoors.

Long-term health risks: Prolonged exposure to VOCs may lead to more serious health problems, including liver, kidney, and central nervous system damage.

Safer Alternatives:

To minimize exposure to these harmful chemicals, consider the following alternatives:

Low-VOC or Zero-VOC Products: Opt for paints, varnishes, and adhesives labeled as low-VOC or zero-VOC. These products emit fewer harmful fumes and are better for indoor air quality.

Formaldehyde-Free Materials: Look for building materials certified as formaldehyde-free or those that use alternative adhesives, such as soy-based resins, that do not emit formaldehyde.

Adequate Ventilation: Ensure proper ventilation during and after the application of paints, varnishes, and installation of materials that may emit VOCs or formaldehyde.

Natural and Non-Toxic Products: Consider using natural products like clay-based paints or natural wood finishes, which are generally free from synthetic chemicals and safer for both health and the environment.

Managing Electronic Waste

Electronic devices such as computers, TVs, and smartphones are complex pieces of technology that incorporate various materials, including heavy metals like lead, cadmium, and mercury. These metals are used for specific purposes within the devices:

1. **Lead:** Historically used in soldering electronic components and in some types of batteries, lead is a potent neurotoxin. Exposure to lead, especially in children, can result in developmental issues, including learning disabilities and behavioral problems. It can also cause neurological damage in adults.
2. **Cadmium:** Found in some types of batteries, semiconductors, and certain types of plastic, cadmium is another neurotoxin. It can accumulate in the body and lead to kidney damage, bone defects, and potentially cancer.
3. **Mercury:** Used in fluorescent lamps and some types of switches, mercury is highly toxic to the nervous system. It can cause cognitive and motor dysfunction, as well as other health issues when exposure occurs.

Batteries are a significant concern because they often contain heavy metals and toxic chemicals. Alkaline batteries, for example, contain manganese, while rechargeable batteries like nickel-cadmium (NiCd) and nickel-metal hydride (NiMH) contain cadmium and rare earth elements, respectively. Lithium-ion batteries, widely used in smartphones and laptops, contain lithium, cobalt, and other metals.

Improper disposal of electronic devices and batteries can lead to environmental contamination. When these items are incinerated or landfilled without proper treatment, the heavy metals and toxic chemicals can leach into the soil and groundwater, posing risks to wildlife and human populations that rely on these water sources. Additionally, when these substances enter the food chain, they can bio accumulate, leading to increased concentrations in higher trophic levels, including humans.

Non-Stick Pans

Composition and Concerns:

Non-stick pans are often coated with polytetrafluoroethylene (PTFE), known as Teflon. Historically, the production of PTFE involved Perfluorooctanoic Acid (PFOA), a man-made chemical.

PFOA is a persistent organic pollutant, meaning it does not break down easily in the environment. It is known to accumulate in the human body and the environment over time.

Health Risks:

Cancer: Some studies have suggested a possible link between PFOA exposure and certain types of cancer, including kidney and testicular cancer.

Thyroid Disease: Exposure to PFOA has been associated with changes in thyroid hormone levels, which can affect metabolism and other bodily functions.

Developmental Problems: PFOA exposure during pregnancy may lead to developmental issues in children, such as low birth weight and altered immune function.

Environmental Impact:

PFOA can be released into the environment during the manufacturing process and when non-stick pans are heated to high temperatures.

It is resistant to degradation, leading to long-term environmental contamination.

Plastic Cutting Boards and Utensils

Composition and Concerns:

Many plastic kitchen items are made with compounds such as Bisphenol A (BPA) and phthalates, which are used to make plastics more durable and flexible.

These chemicals can leach into food, especially when the plastic is exposed to heat or becomes scratched and worn.

Health Risks:

BPA: This chemical can mimic estrogen in the body and has been linked to a range of health issues, including reproductive disorders, heart disease, and increased risk of certain cancers.

Phthalates: These are endocrine disruptors that can interfere with hormone function, potentially leading to reproductive and developmental problems.

Alternatives and Best Practices:

Consider using cookware made from stainless steel, cast iron, or ceramic, which do not contain harmful chemicals.

Choose cutting boards made from materials like wood or bamboo, which are less likely to contain harmful additives.

If using plastic utensils, look for those labeled as BPA-free and avoid exposing them to high temperatures, such as in the microwave or dishwasher.

1. Water-Repellent and Stain-Resistant Fabrics:

Treatment with PFOA: Fabrics designed to repel water and resist stains are often treated with perfluorooctanoic acid (PFOA) or similar compounds known as per- and polyfluoroalkyl substances (PFAS). These chemicals are used because they can create a barrier that prevents liquids from penetrating the fabric.

Health Concerns: PFOA and related chemicals have been associated with several health issues. Research suggests that prolonged exposure can lead to serious conditions such as cancer, thyroid disease, and other endocrine disorders. These compounds are persistent in the environment and in the human body, meaning they do not break down easily and can accumulate over time.

2. Dry-Cleaned Clothing:

Use of Perchloroethylene: Dry cleaning often involves the use of solvents to remove stains and clean fabrics without water. Perchloroethylene, or perc, is a common solvent used in this process.

Health Risks: Perchloroethylene is classified as a probable human carcinogen by the International Agency for Research on Cancer (IARC). Exposure to this chemical can lead to liver and kidney damage and has been linked to an increased risk of certain cancers. People can be exposed through inhalation during the dry-cleaning process or by wearing clothes that have been dry cleaned.

These issues highlight the importance of being aware of the chemicals used in the treatment of clothing and textiles and their potential health impacts. Efforts are being made to find safer alternatives and to increase awareness among consumers about the risks associated with these chemicals. Additionally, some manufacturers are exploring eco-friendly and non-toxic methods for achieving water-repellency and stain resistance.

Health Risks from Furniture and Home Décor

When it comes to furniture and home décor, certain materials and treatments can introduce chemicals into the home environment, which may pose health risks.

Here's a detailed look at the concerns related to upholstered furniture, carpets, and rugs:

1. Upholstered Furniture:

Flame Retardants: These chemicals are added to the foam and fabrics of upholstered furniture to reduce the risk of fire. However, many flame retardants are known endocrine disruptors, which means they can interfere with hormone systems. This interference can lead to reproductive health issues and developmental problems, especially in children.

Formaldehyde: Often used in adhesives and as a finishing agent, formaldehyde is a volatile organic compound (VOC) that can off-gas from furniture over time. It is classified as a known human carcinogen by the International Agency for Research on Cancer (IARC). Exposure to formaldehyde can cause respiratory problems, skin irritation, and has been linked to certain types of cancer.

2. Carpets and Rugs:

VOCs: Carpets and rugs can emit VOCs, which are chemicals that easily become vapors or gases. VOC exposure is associated with a variety of health issues, including headaches, dizziness, and respiratory problems. Long-term exposure can exacerbate these issues, particularly in sensitive individuals such as children and those with asthma.

Flame Retardants and Alkylphenol Ethoxylates (APEs): Like upholstered furniture, carpets and rugs may also contain flame retardants, which can disrupt hormonal systems in the body. APEs are used in the production of textiles and can break down into alkylphenols, which are known endocrine disruptors. These chemicals can affect reproductive health and development.

Overall, the presence of these chemicals in home furnishings highlights the need for increased awareness and consideration of safer alternatives. Consumers can reduce exposure by choosing products labeled as free from harmful chemicals, ensuring proper ventilation in homes, and opting for natural materials when possible. Additionally, manufacturers are increasingly exploring the use of non-toxic substances and sustainable practices in the production of furniture and home décor.

Health Risks from Bleached Paper Products and Thermal Paper Receipts

The use of certain chemicals in the production of paper products can introduce health risks to consumers. Here's a detailed look at the concerns associated with bleached paper towels, napkins, and thermal paper receipts:

1. Bleached Paper Towels and Napkins:

Chlorine and Dioxins: Paper towels and napkins are often bleached to achieve a white appearance. This bleaching process can involve chlorine, this may cause dioxins to be produced as a result. Dioxins are a class of very poisonous chemicals with close chemical relationships to one another and persistent in the environment.

Health Hazards: Dioxins are known to cause a range of serious health issues. They can disrupt reproductive and developmental processes, leading to problems such as infertility and developmental delays in children. Dioxins are also classified as known human carcinogens, meaning they can increase the risk of cancer. Even low-level exposure over time can contribute to these health risks.

2. Receipts and Thermal Paper:

BPA and BPS: Thermal paper, used for printing receipts, often features two substances called bisphenol A (BPA) and bisphenol S (BPS) that are used for develop the ink on the paper through heat.

Health Hazards: One well-known endocrine disruptor is bisphenol A (BPA), which has the ability to imitate the body's hormones and cause endocrine system interference. Hormonal abnormalities, infertility, and an increased chance of developing certain malignancies are among the health concerns that may result from this disturbance particularly breast and prostate cancer. BPS, used as an alternative to BPA, may have similar health effects, while studies are still under progress to determine its complete effects.

The Real Deal on Sanitary Pads: Navigating Chemicals for a Healthier Menstrual Cycle:

Sanitary pads can contain several harmful chemicals that may pose health risks to users. Here are some of the key chemicals and their potential health impacts:

1. **Phthalates**: These chemicals are used to make plastics more flexible and are found in various personal care products. They have been linked to hormone disruption and reproductive issues. Phthalates can affect the reproductive, neurological, and cardiovascular systems.
2. Chemicals known as volatile organic compounds (VOCs) are those that evaporate readily when exposed to room temperature air and can cause respiratory problems and irritation. VOCs have been detected in every brand of sanitary pads tested in a study.
3. **Parabens**: Known for their preservative properties, parabens are used in many personal care products and have been associated with hormone disruption and potential links to breast cancer. Parabens were found in sanitary pads, including organic ones.

4. **Formaldehyde-Releasing Preservatives**: Products are treated with these to stop the development of mold and germs. But formaldehyde is a recognized allergy and carcinogen in and of itself. Adipose tissue was detected in some sanitary pads.
5. **PFAS (Per- and Polyfluoroalkyl Substances)**: These are persistent organic pollutants that are used in various products for their water- and oil-repellent properties. Cancer and reproductive disorders are among the many health concerns associated with PFAS. PFAS were found in 48% of sanitary pads tested.
6. **Dioxins**: Although primarily associated with tampons, dioxins can also be present in sanitary pads, especially if the cotton used in the pads is bleached. Dioxins are known to cause cancer and hormone disruption.
7. **Pesticide Residues**: If the cotton used in the pads is not organically grown, it may contain pesticide residues, which can be harmful to health, especially if the pads come into contact with sensitive skin.
8. **Fragrance**: The fragrance in sanitary pads can contain a variety of chemicals, including allergens, sensitizers, and neurotoxins, which can cause skin irritation and other health issues .

These chemicals can potentially lead to health issues such as hormone disruption, reproductive problems, skin irritation, and even cancer. It is important for consumers to be aware of these potential risks and consider using products that are free from harmful chemicals.

Best Practices for Storing Food to Minimize Chemical Leaching

Food packaging is an important aspect of food safety and preservation, but it can also be a source of harmful chemical exposure. Here's a deeper look into the issues related to canned foods and plastic wraps and bags:

1. **Canned Foods**:
   BPA in Can Linings: Bisphenol A (BPA) is commonly used in the epoxy resins that line metal cans to prevent corrosion and contamination of the food by the metal. However, BPA can leach into the food, especially when the cans are heated or stored for long periods.
   Health Risks: BPA is an endocrine disruptor, meaning it can interfere with the body's hormone systems. This can lead to a variety of health issues, including hormonal imbalances, reproductive problems, and an increased risk of certain cancers, such as breast and prostate cancer. Additionally, exposure to BPA has been linked to heart disease, diabetes, and developmental issues in children.

2. **Plastic Wraps and Bags**:
   Phthalates and Plasticizers: These chemicals are often used in plastic wraps and bags to make them flexible and durable. Phthalates can migrate from the packaging into the food, especially when the plastic is heated or comes into contact with fatty foods.

Health Risks: Phthalates are also endocrine disruptors and have been associated with hormonal imbalances, reproductive health issues, and developmental problems in children. Prolonged exposure can have wide-ranging effects, including impacts on fertility and the potential for increased risk of certain chronic health conditions.

To minimize exposure to these chemicals, consumers can take several steps:

Choose BPA-Free Products: Look for canned goods labeled as BPA-free or opt for products packaged in glass or cardboard.

Use Glass or Stainless Steel Containers: For food storage, consider using glass or stainless steel containers instead of plastic to avoid chemical leaching.

Mindful Product Choices: Avoid plastic wraps and bags for prolonged storage, especially with fatty or acidic foods. Consider alternatives like beeswax wraps or silicone covers.

Natural Alternatives: Use natural cleaning products and personal care items to reduce exposure to harmful chemicals.

Sustainable Practices: Proper disposal and recycling of electronic devices and batteries can help reduce environmental contamination and protect overall health.

Exposure to harmful chemicals in everyday products is a significant concern, as it can lead to a broad range of health risks. Here's an in-depth look at these risks and strategies to minimize exposure:

Health Risks from Chemical Exposure:

1. **Reproductive and Developmental Issues:**
   Chemicals Involved: Phthalates and BPA are common offenders.
   Effects: These chemicals can disrupt hormones, potentially leading to fertility problems, developmental issues in children, and an increased risk of birth defects.
2. **Cancer:**
   Chemicals Involved: Formaldehyde and certain VOCs (Volatile Organic Compounds) are known or suspected carcinogens.
   Effects: Long-term exposure can increase cancer risk, affecting various organs depending on the chemical.
3. **Endocrine Disruption:**
   Chemicals Involved: Endocrine-disrupting chemicals like BPA interfere with the hormonal system.
   Effects: This can lead to metabolic disorders, obesity, diabetes, and other hormonal imbalances.
4. **Respiratory Problems:**
   Chemicals Involved: Formaldehyde and some VOCs can irritate the respiratory tract.
   Effects: This can cause coughing, wheezing, and in severe cases, contribute to chronic respiratory diseases.
5. **Neurological Effects:**
   Chemicals Involved: Heavy metals like lead and mercury are particularly harmful.
   Effects: They can cause neurological damage, cognitive impairment, and behavioral issues, especially in children.

6. **Skin and Eye Irritation**:
   Chemicals Involved: Many household chemicals can cause irritation.
   Effects: Contact with the skin or eyes can lead to dermatitis, allergic reactions, or irritation.
7. **Immune System Suppression**:
   Chemicals Involved: Certain toxic substances may weaken immunity.
   Effects: Because of this, people may get sick more easily.
8. **Cardiovascular Issues**:
   Chemicals Involved: Exposure to some chemicals has been linked to heart problems.
   Effects: It can increase the risk of cardiovascular diseases, including hypertension and heart disease.
9. **Liver and Kidney Damage**:
   Chemicals Involved: Prolonged exposure to toxic substances can harm these organs.
   Effects: This can impair their ability to detoxify the body and perform essential functions.
10. **Thyroid Dysfunction**:
    Chemicals Involved: Chemicals like PFOA can affect thyroid function.
    Effects: This can lead to hypothyroidism or hyperthyroidism, with various health consequences.

Strategies to Minimize Exposure:

1. **Read Labels Carefully**:
   Look for products labeled BPA-free, phthalate-free, and paraben-free.

Be cautious of terms like "natural" or "green," which may not guarantee safety.

2. **Opt for Glass or Stainless Steel**:
Use these materials for food storage and water bottles to avoid chemical leaching from plastics.

3. **Avoid Heating Plastic**:
Do not microwave food in plastic containers.
Avoid using plastic for hot drinks.

4. **Use Natural Cleaning Products**:
Make DIY cleaners using vinegar, baking soda, and lemon juice.
Choose commercial products free of VOCs, ammonia, and chlorine.

5. **Be Mindful of Personal Care Products**:
Check ingredient lists for harmful substances like parabens and phthalates.
Opt for products certified by organizations such as the Environmental Working Group (EWG).
Open windows and use exhaust fans to make sure there is enough ventilation to reduce indoor air pollution from VOCs.

6. **Choose Organic Textiles**:
Opt for organic clothing and bedding to avoid chemicals like flame retardants and formaldehyde.

7. **Limit Dry Cleaning**:
Choose washable fabrics or air out dry-cleaned items before use.

8. **Dispose of Electronics and Batteries Properly**:
Use recycling programs to prevent environmental contamination.

9. **Filter Your Water**:
   Install home filtration systems to remove contaminants. Choose BPA-free bottled water brands.
10. **Use Safe Cookware**:
    Prefer stainless steel, cast iron, or ceramic cookware over non-stick pans containing PFOA.
11. **Stay Informed and Educated**:
    Use resources like the EWG's Skin Deep database to research products.
12. **Advocate for Safer Products**:
    Support legislation regulating harmful chemicals. Choose brands that prioritize health and safety.

3

TOXIC-FREE TASTE

*M*odern cookware can pose hidden dangers, such as nonstick cookware, which releases toxic fumes when overheated and often contains PFAS linked to health issues. Aluminum cookware can leach aluminum into food, potentially associated with neurodegenerative diseases. Unlined copper cookware can cause toxicity by leaching copper into food, while some ceramic cookware may contain lead or cadmium in the glaze, potentially leaching if damaged. Cast iron cookware can leach excessive iron, posing a risk for individuals with high iron levels. Awareness of these risks helps in making informed and safe cookware choices.

Nonstick pan:

A nonstick pan is typically made up of a metal base, often aluminum or stainless steel, coated with a nonstick material that prevents food from sticking to the surface. The most common nonstick coating is polytetrafluoroethylene (PTFE), most people associate it with the brand Teflon. Polytetrafluoroethylene (PTFE) is an artificial fluid fluoropolymer that has excellent nonstick properties and is resistant to high temperatures, making it ideal for cookware.

Side Effects and Concerns:

1. **Chemical Exposure**: Chemical exposure is a major worry when it comes to nonstick cookware. When nonstick pans are heated to high temperatures, typically above 500°F (260°C), they can release toxic fumes called perfluorooctanoic acid (PFOA) and other fluorinated compounds. These fumes can be harmful to humans and are particularly dangerous to birds, which can die from inhaling them.
2. **Scratching and Flaking**: Nonstick coatings can scratch and flake over time, especially with the use of metal utensils or abrasive cleaners. This can lead to ingestion of the nonstick material, which is not considered safe if it enters the body.
3. **Environmental Concerns**: The production and disposal of nonstick cookware raise environmental concerns. PFOA, which was used in the production of PTFE, is a persistent organic pollutant that does not break down easily in the environment. It has been linked to various health issues in humans and animals. Due to these concerns, many manufacturers have phased out the use of PFOA in their products.
4. **Heat Limitations**: Nonstick pans are not suitable for searing and stir-frying, both of which use high temperatures, may damage the nonstick coating. This can limit the versatility of the cookware.
5. **Durability**: Nonstick pans usually don't last as long as other kinds of cookware. The nonstick surface can degrade over time, reducing the effectiveness of the pan and potentially leading to the need for more frequent replacements.

It's important to note that while there are concerns associated with nonstick cookware, many people use it safely by following guidelines such as avoiding high-heat cooking, using wooden or plastic utensils to prevent scratching, and replacing pans when the nonstick surface starts to degrade. Additionally, there are alternative nonstick materials available, such as ceramic or diamond-infused coatings, which may have different safety profiles and environmental impacts.

Practical Tips for Safe Use:

➤ Avoid overheating Teflon pans by cooking on low to medium heat.
➤ Ensure proper ventilation to disperse any fumes.
➤ Discard cookware showing signs of degradation, such as scratches or flaking.
➤ Teflon's convenience comes with potential health risks due to toxic fume release and long-term health issues linked to PFOA exposure.
➤ Safer alternatives like stainless steel, cast iron, and ceramic-coated cookware are available.
➤ Practical steps can minimize risks for those continuing to use Teflon cookware.
➤ By staying informed and making conscious choices, consumers can enjoy the benefits of non-stick cookware while prioritizing their health and safety.

Aluminum cookware:

Cooking in aluminum cookware has been a subject of concern due to potential health hazards associated with the leaching of aluminum into food. Aluminum is a reactive metal, and under certain conditions, it can dissolve into the food being cooked, potentially leading to health issues. Here are some of the health hazards associated with cooking in aluminum, along with reasons and references:

1. **Neurological Disorders:** Aluminum has been linked to neurological disorders, particularly Alzheimer's disease. Some studies suggest that the accumulation of aluminum in the brain may contribute to the formation of neurofibrillary tangles, which are a hallmark of Alzheimer's pathology.
   Reference: "Aluminum and Alzheimer's disease: after a century of controversy, is there a plausible link?" by Exley, C., Journal of Alzheimer's Disease, 2014.
2. **Bone Health:** Aluminum can interfere with calcium and phosphorus metabolism, potentially leading to bone disorders. It can accumulate in bones and may contribute to the development of osteoporosis or other bone-related conditions.
3. **Kidney Damage:** Individuals with kidney disorders are particularly at risk from aluminum exposure because their bodies cannot effectively excrete the metal. Aluminum accumulation can lead to further kidney damage and bone disease in these patients.
4. **Acidic Foods:** Cooking acidic foods (such as tomato sauce, citrus fruits, and vinegar) in aluminum cookware can cause the metal to leach into the food at higher rates. This is because acids can react with aluminum, leading to increased dissolution.
5. **Antacids and Acid Blockers:** People who consume antacids or acid blockers may be at increased risk of aluminum toxicity

because these medications can increase the gastrointestinal absorption of aluminum.

It's important to note that the overall risk of aluminum toxicity from cooking in aluminum cookware is generally considered low for healthy individuals. The body has mechanisms to regulate and excrete aluminum, and the amounts typically leached into food are not usually significant enough to cause harm. However, people with certain health conditions, such as kidney disease, or those who are exposed to high levels of aluminum from multiple sources, may be at greater risk.

To minimize potential exposure, some people choose to use alternative cookware materials such as stainless steel, cast iron, or non-stick coatings. When using aluminum cookware, it's advisable to avoid cooking highly acidic or salty foods for extended periods and to avoid using abrasive cleaners that can scratch the surface, potentially increasing the leaching of aluminum.

Cast Iron

Seasoning: Proper seasoning is key to maintaining the surface that won't stick. Coat the pan with a thin layer of oil and cook it in the oven to season it oven to create a natural, polymerized oil coating.

Maintenance: Avoid using soap to clean cast iron as it can strip the seasoning. Instead, rinse with hot water and a stiff brush, then dry thoroughly and re-oil lightly.

Cooking Tips: Preheat the pan slowly to prevent warping and always use a lower heat setting than you would with non-stick pans.

Stainless Steel

Heat Distribution: Stainless steel pans can have hot spots, so it's important to use them on medium heat and stir or flip food regularly.

Stickiness: Food can stick to stainless steel, especially if it's not properly preheated. To prevent sticking, heat the pan first, add oil, and let it heat up before adding food.

Cleaning: Stainless steel can discolor or develop a rainbow tint if overheated. Clean with a non-abrasive sponge or stainless-steel cleaner to maintain its appearance.

Ceramic Cookware

Quality: As you mentioned, it's crucial to choose high-quality ceramic cookware. Look for products that are free from lead, cadmium, and other harmful substances.

Heat Limitations: Ceramic pans are generally less heat-resistant than cast iron or stainless steel. Avoid using them at very high temperatures to prevent the non-stick coating from degrading.

Care: Avoid using metal utensils with ceramic pots and pans, as they might abrade the surface and diminish the non-stick properties.

General Precautions

Temperature Control: No matter what kind of cookware you use, you should never let your pans become too hot. High temperatures can not only damage the cookware but also increase the risk of harmful chemical release, especially with non-stick pans.

Ventilation: Ensure good kitchen ventilation when cooking, as some cookware and cooking methods can release fumes, especially when heated to high temperatures.

Lifecycle Consideration: Consider the entire lifecycle of your cookware, from production to disposal. Opting for durable, long-lasting materials like cast iron or stainless steel can reduce waste and environmental impact.

Mud vessel:

Using mud vessels, also known as earthenware or terracotta pots, for cooking is a traditional practice that has been is making a comeback because to the positive effects it has on health and the environment. It is important to note the following things about using mud vessels for cooking:

Benefits of Mud Vessels

Healthy Cooking: Mud vessels are made from natural clay, which is free from chemicals and toxins. Cooking in mud vessels can help retain the nutritional value of food, as they do not leach harmful substances into the food.

Moisture Retention: These pots are porous, which allows them to absorb and release moisture. This helps in retaining the moisture content of the food, making it softer and more flavorful.

Even Heat Distribution: Mud vessels distribute heat evenly, which is ideal for slow cooking. This can help in breaking breaks down the resistant fibers in food, facilitating digestion.

Environmentally Friendly: Clay is a natural and sustainable material. Mud vessels are biodegradable in comparison to synthetic or metal alternatives, and they are easier on the environment cookware.

Precautions and Tips

Seasoning: Similar to cast iron, mud vessels need to be seasoned before first use. This involves soaking the pot in water for several hours to remove any impurities and to prevent cracking during cooking.

Gradual Heating: Always heat mud vessels gradually to prevent them from cracking. Bring the temperature up to the appropriate level slowly at first.

Avoid Extreme Temperature Changes: Do not place a hot mud vessel directly into cold water or vice versa, as this can cause it to crack.

Cleaning: Clean mud vessels using a gentle sponge and warm water. Stay away from soap, as it can absorb into the porous clay. Do not use metal scrubbers, as they can scratch the surface.

Storage: Store mud vessels in a dry place to prevent mold growth. If not used for an extended re-seasoning them before usage is a good idea, period.

Cooking Tips

Slow Cooking: Mud vessels are ideal for slow cooking methods like stews, soups, and curries. They help in infusing the food with flavors and aromas.

Water Content: Add a little extra water when cooking in mud vessels, as they tend to absorb some moisture.

Lid Placement: Use a tight-fitting lid to trap the steam and moisture inside, which helps in faster cooking and better flavor retention.

Environmental Considerations

Sustainability: Opting for mud vessels supports sustainable and traditional craftsmanship. They are a renewable resource they produce less waste when compared to synthetic or metal alternatives cookware.

Local Artisans: Purchasing mud vessels from local artisans can help support traditional skills and contribute to local economies.

By using mud vessels for cooking, you not only enjoy improve the quality of our food while also making a positive impact on the environment. But be careful while handling and maintaining these boats so their longevity and effectiveness.

4

DIGITAL DILEMMAS

Introduction

In the modern world, electronic gadgets such as smartphones, tablets, laptops, as well as other electronic gadgets now play an essential role in our everyday life. Although these technologies provide a plethora of advantages, such as accessibility, ease, and connectedness to information, they also pose potential health risks. This documentary delves into the various health issues that can arise from prolonged and improper use of electronic gadgets, exploring consequences on the neurological system, eyesight, psychological well-being, and other areas.

Problems with the Nervous System and Magnetic Fields

Technology has become an integral part of our everyday lives that the potential health implications of their electromagnetic fields (EMFs) often go unnoticed. Yet, understanding their impact on the nervous system is crucial. Let's explore how these fields might affect us:

Magnetic Fields (EMFs)

Electronic gadgets are surrounded by electromagnetic fields, which are regions of energy. Computers, Wi-Fi routers, mobile phones, and other wireless devices are the sources of these fields. While EMFs are a natural part of the environment, the artificial EMFs created by these gadgets have raised health concerns.

Potential Effects on the Nervous System

1. **Nerve Function:**

   EMFs can potentially interfere with the electrical activity of neurons, the cells responsible for transmitting signals in the nervous system. This interference could disrupt normal nerve function, possibly leading to symptoms such as tingling, numbness, or even more severe neurological disturbances over time.

   Some studies suggest that EMF exposure may alter the permeability of the blood-brain barrier, which protects the brain from harmful substances. This could potentially lead to neurological damage or disease.

2. **Headaches and Sleep Disturbances:**

   Frequent exposure to EMFs has been associated with headaches and migraines. The exact mechanism is not fully understood, but it is thought that EMFs could affect neurotransmitter release or neural excitability, leading to pain.

   Sleep disturbances are another common complaint. EMFs can interfere with melatonin production, a hormone that regulates sleep cycles. This disruption can lead to insomnia or poor-quality sleep, which might contribute to chronic fatigue and mood disorders.

3. **Neurological Disorders:**
   There is ongoing research into the potential link between long-term EMF exposure and neurological disorders. Some studies have suggested that chronic exposure could increase the risk of diseases like Alzheimer's or Parkinson's by promoting oxidative stress and inflammation in neural tissues.

While these links are not yet definitively proven, they underscore the importance of further research to understand the long-term implications of EMF exposure.

Mitigation Strategies

Given these potential risks, several strategies can help mitigate EMF exposure from electronic gadgets:

Limiting Device Use: Reducing the time spent on electronic devices can decrease overall EMF exposure.

Distance: Keeping devices at a distance (e.g., using speakerphone or earphones for calls) can reduce exposure.

Sleep Environment: Keeping gadgets out of the bedroom can minimize nighttime exposure, promoting better sleep.

Awareness and Education: Understanding the potential risks and promoting further research are essential for public health.

Cancer Risks and Radiofrequency Radiation

The potential link between mobile phone radiation and cancer has been a subject of scientific investigation and public concern for many years. Here's a detailed exploration of the issue, along with references to key studies and reports:

Radiofrequency (RF) Radiation

RF radiation is a type of non-ionizing electromagnetic radiation emitted by wireless devices such as mobile phones, tablets, and Wi-Fi routers. Unlike ionizing radiation (e.g., X-rays), which can remove tightly bound electrons from atoms, non-ionizing radiation lacks sufficient energy to cause such ionization but can still have biological effects.

Potential Mechanism of Risk

1. **Absorption by Tissues:**
   When a mobile phone is used, RF radiation is absorbed by the tissues closest to where the device is held, such as the head and neck. The concern is that this absorption could potentially lead to changes at the cellular level, such as DNA damage, which might contribute to cancer development.
2. **IARC Classification:**
   The International Agency for Research on Cancer (IARC), part of the World Health Organization (WHO), has classified RF electromagnetic fields as "possibly carcinogenic to humans" (Group 2B). This classification was based on an increased risk for glioma, a malignant type of brain cancer, observed in some epidemiological studies. The IARC concluded that there was limited evidence in humans and animals but enough to warrant caution

1. **Key Studies and Reports**

INTERPHONE Study: The INTERPHONE study, a large international case-control study, investigated the potential link between mobile phone use and brain tumors. It found a slight increase in the risk of glioma in the highest category of cumulative call time, but the authors noted potential biases and errors that prevent a causal interpretation.

Danish Cohort Study: This study followed a large cohort of mobile phone subscribers in Denmark and found no increased risk of brain tumors associated with mobile phone use. However, the study's methodology has been critiqued, particularly regarding its classification of mobile phone users.

U.S. National Toxicology Program (NTP) Studies: The NTP conducted animal studies to assess the cancer risk from RF radiation. The studies found some evidence of an increased risk of certain types of tumors in male rats exposed to high levels of RF radiation similar to those used in mobile communications.

Recommendations to Mitigate Risks

While definitive causal links between RF radiation and cancer have not been established, precautionary measures are recommended:

Use Speakerphones or Earphones: Keeping the phone away from the head reduces RF exposure.

Limit Call Duration: Reducing the time spent on calls can decrease exposure.

Text Instead of Call: Sending text messages instead of making voice calls can further reduce exposure.

Use Airplane Mode: When not actively using the device, keeping it on airplane mode can minimize radiation emission.

While the evidence linking RF radiation from mobile phones to cancer is not conclusive, ongoing research continues to investigate this potential risk. It is prudent to follow recommended precautions to minimize exposure while awaiting more definitive scientific findings.

Vision Problems and Digital Eye Strain

The increasing use of electronic devices in daily life has brought about a rise in vision-related issues, commonly referred to as Digital Eye Strain or Computer Vision Syndrome. Let's explore these issues in detail, along with references to key studies and reports:

Symptoms and Causes of Digital Eye Strain

1. **Symptoms:**
   Users often experience eye fatigue, dryness, irritation, difficulty focusing, and headaches. These symptoms can significantly impact comfort and productivity, especially when using screens for extended periods.
2. **Contributing Factors:**
   Poor Lighting and Glare: Inadequate ambient lighting and glare from screens can exacerbate eye strain. Adjusting screen brightness and positioning screens to avoid glare can help alleviate symptoms.

Improper Viewing Distances: Sitting too close or too far from the screen can lead to strain. The ideal viewing distance is typically about an arm's length away.

Uncorrected Vision Problems: Uncorrected refractive errors can intensify symptoms. Regular eye exams and proper corrective lenses are essential.

Impact of Blue Light

The blue light emitted by digital screens is a particular concern because it can penetrate deep into the eye, potentially causing retinal damage. Prolonged exposure to blue light has been linked to:

Retinal Damage: Some studies suggest that excessive blue light exposure may contribute to retinal damage and increase the risk of age-related macular degeneration.

Sleep Disturbances: Blue light can interfere with melatonin production, disrupting sleep patterns and leading to insomnia or poor sleep quality.

Recommendations and Mitigation Strategies

1. **The 20-20-20 Rule:**
   Many people find that following the 20-20-20 rule helps them deal with digital eye strain. This requires you to glance at anything 20 feet away for 20 seconds every 20 minutes. Reducing weariness and tension in the eyes is one benefit of this technique.
2. **Screen Adjustments:**
   Adjusting the screen's brightness and contrast to comfortable levels can reduce glare and strain. Using screen filters to block blue light is also beneficial.
3. **Work Environment:**

Improving work environment ergonomics can help, such as adjusting chair height, ensuring proper screen height, and using anti-glare screens.

5

BEHAVIORAL AND CHARACTER CHANGES AND EXCESSIVE ELECTRONIC GADGET USE

The widespread use of electronic gadgets among children and adolescents is linked to significant behavioral and character changes. These changes are a growing concern, given the increasing accessibility and allure of digital media. Here's a detailed exploration of these issues, supported by studies and reports:

Impact on Attention and Academic Performance

1. **Reduced Attention Span:**
   The fast-paced and interactive nature of digital content, especially on social media and gaming platforms, can lead

to reduced attention spans in children and adolescents. This constant stimulation can make it hard for kids to concentrate on boring activities, such as studying or reading, which require sustained attention.

2. **Poor Academic Performance:**
Excessive gadget use often correlates with poorer academic outcomes. A study found that students who excessively use electronic devices tend to have lower grades, primarily due to distractions and reduced study time.

Social Interaction and Mental Health

1. **Impaired Social Interactions:**
Overuse of gadgets can lead to impaired social skills, as children might prefer interacting online rather than in person. This preference can hinder the development of essential social and communication skills, which are crucial during formative years.

2. **Increased Anxiety and Depression:**
Overexposure to digital content and online interactions associated with increased teenage stress, despair, and irritability. The pressure to maintain a certain online persona and the fear of missing out (FOMO) can exacerbate these issues

Addiction and Brain Chemistry

1. **Digital Addiction:**
The addictive nature of social media and gaming platforms is well-documented. These platforms are designed to provide instant gratification, which can lead to addictive behaviors, similar to substance addiction. This addiction can alter brain

chemistry, affecting reward pathways and impacting emotional regulations.

2. **Altered Brain Development:**
Continuous exposure to digital media during critical developmental periods can have long-term effects on brain development. The overstimulation provided by gadgets can affect the development of neural circuits involved in attention, impulse control, and decision-making.

Mitigation Strategies

➢ **Balanced Use:**

Encouraging balanced gadget use is crucial. In order to lessen the impact, it is recommended to promote offline activities and set limitations on screen usage.

➢ **Promote Offline Activities:**

Encouraging participation in sports, hobbies, and social activities can help develop social skills and reduce dependency on gadgets.

➢ **Parental Monitoring and Guidance:**

Parents and guardians can play a vital role by monitoring usage, setting boundaries, and ensuring that digital content is age-appropriate.

Cardiovascular and Heart Problems Related to Gadget Use

The modern lifestyle, characterized by extensive use of electronic gadgets, has contributed to an increase in sedentary behavior, which is a significant risk factor for cardiovascular and heart problems. Here's an in-depth look at how gadget use can impact heart health and strategies to mitigate these effects:

Impact of Sedentary Lifestyle on Cardiovascular Health

1. **Prolonged Sitting and Physical Inactivity:**
   Extended periods of sitting while using electronic devices can lead to a range of cardiovascular issues. Physical inactivity increases the likelihood of being overweight, hypertensive, and suffering from cardiovascular disease. Inactivity lowers blood flow, which increases the risk of atherosclerosis (the development of fatty deposits in the arteries) and cardiovascular disease (heart attacks and strokes).

2. **Metabolic Syndrome and Obesity Syndrome:**
   Sedentary behavior contributes leading to obesity and excess weight, which greatly increase the likelihood of cardiovascular diseases. Obesity often leads to An elevated risk of cardiovascular disease is exacerbated by metabolic syndrome, a collection of symptoms includes hypertension, diabetes, abdominal obesity, and abnormal cholesterol levels.

Stress in the Mind and the Heart Health

1. **Stress and Anxiety from Connectivity:**
   The constant connectivity enabled by gadgets can lead to information overload, stress, and anxiety. This psychological stress can elevate cortisol levels, a hormone that, when chronically elevated, could lead to hypertension, insomnia, and cardiovascular disease.

2. **Impact of Cortisol:**
   When cortisol levels are high, people tend to eat more and want items that are rich in calories, contributing to weight gain. Cortisol also affects how the body metabolizes fats, carbohydrates, and proteins, potentially leading to increased risk factors for cardiovascular diseases.

Mitigation Strategies for Heart Health

1. **Incorporating Physical Activity:**
   Engaging in regular physical activity is crucial for countering the effects of a sedentary lifestyle. Even moderate exercise, such as walking, cycling, or swimming, can improve circulation, reduce weight, and lower blood pressure, thereby reducing the risk of heart disease
2. **Taking Frequent Breaks:**
   Taking regular breaks from sitting can help improve circulation lower the risk of heart issues. Regular physical activity, such as standing, stretching, or going for brief walks every hour can make a significant difference.

Reducing Stress with Mindfulness Practices:

Meditation and deep breathing exercises are all examples of mindfulness activities that may help manage stress and lessen the harmful effects of cortisol on heart health. These routines help you unwind and may lead to better control of blood pressure and heart rates.

6

MINDFUL EATING

*U*sing electronic gadgets during meals has become a common habit for many people, but it can negatively impact digestive health. Let's explore how this behavior affects digestion and what can be done to mitigate these effects:

Impact of Distracted Eating on Digestion

1. **Overeating and Poor Chewing:**
   When individuals use gadgets during meals, they are more likely to eat mindlessly, paying less attention to portion sizes and satiety cues. Distracted eating often leads to overeating because people are less aware of how much they are consuming. Additionally, they may not chew their food thoroughly, which is the first crucial step in the digestive process
2. **Disruption of Digestive Processes:**
   Poor chewing can lead to larger food particles entering the gastrointestinal tract, reducing the efficiency with which food is broken down by the stomach and intestines. This can result in digestive discomfort, such as bloating and gas. Moreover,

overeating can cause the stomach to produce excess acid, leading to acid reflux or heartburn

3. **Risk of Irritable Bowel Syndrome (IBS):**
   While distracted eating itself may not directly cause IBS, it can exacerbate symptoms in individuals who are predisposed to the condition. The stress and hurried eating associated with using gadgets during meals Poo, gas, and other irritable bowel syndrome symptoms may be brought on by or intensified by certain foods.

Benefits of Mindful Eating

1. **Focus on the Meal:**
   Mindful eating involves paying full attention to the experience of eating—savoring the taste, texture, and aroma of the food. By focusing on the meal without distractions, individuals can better recognize their body's hunger and fullness cues, which helps prevent overeating.
2. **Improved Digestion:**
   Taking the time to chew food properly and eat slowly allows the digestive system to function more effectively. Thorough chewing breaks down food into smaller particles, easing the digestive workload on the stomach and intestines and improving nutrient absorption
3. **Reduced Digestive Discomfort:**
   Mindful eating can reduce symptoms of digestive discomfort, such as bloating and acid reflux. By giving the digestive system time to process food at a natural pace, the risk of overproduction of stomach acid and subsequent reflux is minimized

Practical Tips for Mindful Eating

Set the Scene: Create a pleasant eating environment by setting the table and eliminating distractions like phones, TVs, and computers.

Eat Slowly: Take small bites and chew thoroughly, savoring each mouthful.

Listen to Your Body: Pay attention to hunger and satiety signals, stopping when you feel comfortably full.

Engage Your Senses: Notice the colors, smells, and textures of your food to enhance the eating experience.

While electronic gadgets have made life more convenient and connected, it is essential to be aware of their potential health impacts. Adopting healthier usage habits such as setting screen time limits, ensuring ergonomic setups, taking regular breaks, and engaging in physical activities—can help mitigate these risks. Continuous research and public awareness are crucial in understanding and balancing the benefits and challenges of our digital lives.

7

THE EFFECTS OF PESTICIDES ON ECOSYSTEMS AND PEOPLE

$\mathcal{P}$esticides are chemicals that farmers employ to keep unwanted creatures out of their fields, grocery shops, and houses. Chemicals including pesticides, herbicides, rodenticides, and fungicides are all part of this category each designed to target specific pests.

Types of Pesticides

Pesticides are broadly categorized based on the type of pest they are designed to control. Each category targets specific pests to protect crops, food stores, and homes. Below is an elaboration on the main types of pesticides:

1. Insecticides

Definition:

Insecticides are pesticides specifically formulated to control insects and their eggs. They are crucial in reducing the destruction and contamination of crops caused by insect pests.

Mechanism of Action: To kill or paralyze insects, insecticides wreak havoc on their neurological systems. To further restrict the insect's ability to reproduce, certain pesticides aim directly at the insect's reproductive organs hatching of larvae.

Examples:

Organophosphates: Such as chlorpyrifos, which has been restricted or banned in many countries due to its toxicity.

Carbamates: Like carbaryl, which is less toxic than organophosphates and breaks down more quickly in the environment.

Pyrethroids: Synthetic versions of the natural insecticide found in chrysanthemums, such as deltamethrin.

Neonicotinoids: These are a newer class of insecticides, like imidacloprid, which are highly effective however their effects on pollinators like bees have prompted others to express worry.

Usage:

Insecticides are applied to crops, stored grains, and household environments to manage a broad variety of mosquitoes, flies, moths, and beetles as pests.

2. Herbicides (Weed Killers)

Definition:

Herbicides are chemicals used to control or kill weeds. They are essential for improving crop yields by eliminating competition for nutrients, water, and sunlight.

Mechanism of Action: Herbicides can act in several ways, including inhibiting photosynthesis, disrupting plant growth hormones, or blocking the synthesis of essential amino acids.

Examples:

Glyphosate: A broad-spectrum herbicide known by the brand name Roundup, which is used to control weeds in both agricultural and non-agricultural settings.

2,4-D is a selective herbicide that is applied to cereal crops in order to reduce broadleaf weeds.

Dicamba: For use in weed management among cotton and soybean crops.

Usage:

Herbicides are applied to fields before or after planting to control weeds, and they are also used in lawns, gardens, and along roadsides.

3. Rodenticides

Definition:

Rodenticides are pesticides designed to control rodents such as rats and mice. They are important for preventing the destruction of crops and the spread of rodent-borne diseases.

Mechanism of Action: Rodenticides can be either acute (fast-acting) or chronic (slow-acting). Acute rodenticides cause rapid death, while chronic rodenticides are designed to be consumed over time, leading to the death of the rodent.

Examples:

Anticoagulants: Such as warfarin, which prevent blood clotting, leading to internal bleeding and death.

Cholecalciferol (Vitamin D3): Causes hypercalcemia in rodents, leading to kidney failure.

Bromethalin: Affects the central rodents' neurological systems, resulting in death by paralysis.

Usage:

Pesticides are used in agricultural settings, food storage facilities, and residential areas to control rodent populations.

4. Fungicides

Definition:

Fungicides are pesticides used to control fungal diseases in crops and seeds. In order to prevent fungal rot and other fungal illnesses, they play an essential role in safeguarding harvested crops and seeds.

Mechanism of Action: In order to prevent fungus from multiplying, fungicides may damage fungal cell walls and interfere with their energy production, or blocking spore production.

Examples:

Copper Fungicides: Such as copper sulfate, It is used for the management of certain fungal illnesses.

Dithiocarbamates: Like mancozeb, which protect plants from various fungal pathogens.

Triazoles: Such as tebuconazole, in order to prevent cereal crop fungal infections.

Usage:

Fungicides are applied to crops before and after harvest to prevent fungal infections that can reduce crop quality and yield.

Each type of pesticide plays a critical role in modern agriculture and pest management. Insecticides protect crops from insect damage, herbicides improve crop yields by controlling weeds, rodenticides prevent the spread of rodent-borne diseases, and fungicides prevent fungal rot on seeds and crops. Despite their usefulness, pesticides pose serious risks to both humans and the environment if not handled properly.

Artificial Herbicides:

The chemical formulas of synthetic insecticides are industrial laboratories to provide stability, a long shelf life, and ease of distribution. They are designed to be highly effective against target pests while minimizing harm to ecosystems and non-target species. However, the balance between efficacy and safety is challenging, and some synthetic pesticides have faced restrictions or bans due to their environmental and health impacts.

Below is an elaboration on the major classes of **synthetic pesticides:**

1. Organophosphates

Definition:

Organophosphates are a class of insecticides that attack the insects' neurological systems. To do this, they block the enzyme acetylcholinesterase an enzyme essential for nerve function, leading to overstimulation of the nervous system and eventually death.

Examples:

Chlorpyrifos: Used against a wide range of insect pests, such as fleas, mosquitoes, and termites. It is now against the law in several countries due to its toxicity and potential to cause neurological damage.

Parathion: Used on crops like cotton, corn, and fruit trees. Improper handling might result in serious poisoning due to its high toxicity.

Toxicity Concerns:

Organophosphates can be highly toxic to humans and wildlife. Some studies have connected them to neurological diseases, issues with children's development, and other health issues. Due to these concerns, many organophosphates have been restricted or banned in various parts of the world.

2. Carbamates

Definition:

Carbamates are another class of insecticides that act on the nervous system by inhibiting acetylcholinesterase. However, they are generally considered less toxic than organophosphates because their effects are more reversible and tend to wear off more quickly.

Examples:

Carbaryl (Sevin): Used for the control of many insect pests that attack fruits, vegetables, and other crops ornamental plants.

Aldicarb: Used on crops like cotton, potatoes, and watermelons. It is highly toxic to humans and has been banned in several countries.

Toxicity Concerns:

While less toxic than organophosphates, carbamates can still endanger the health of those involved in farming as well as consumers in the absence of adequate management of residues. They can cause symptoms like nausea, headache, and muscle twitching.

3. Pyrethroids

Definition:

Pyrethroids are synthetic versions of the natural insecticide found in chrysanthemum flowers. They are designed to mimic the insecticidal properties of pyrethrins, which are the active compounds in the flowers.

Examples:

Deltamethrin: Used against a variety of insect pests, including mosquitoes, fleas, and ticks.

Permethrin: Used on crops and in household products to control insects like ants, cockroaches, and fleas.

Toxicity Concerns:

Pyrethroids are generally considered to have low toxicity to humans and are often used as a safer alternative to organophosphates and carbamates. However, they can be toxic to aquatic organisms and some beneficial insects like bees.

4. Organochlorines

Definition:

Organochlorines are a class of pesticides that were widely used in the mid-20th century. They are characterized by their persistence in nature and their potential to build up in the food web.

Examples:

DDT (Dichlorodiphenyltrichloroethane): Famous for its use in controlling mosquitoes and other insect pests. It has been banned in many countries due to its environmental persistence and bioaccumulation.

Lindane: Used to control insects on crops and as a treatment for lice and scabies. It has been restricted or banned in many countries due to its toxicity and environmental impact.

Toxicity Concerns:

Organochlorines are associated with an array of medical conditions, including as cancer, infertility, and disturbances to the endocrine system. They bioaccumulate in animal tissues and are persistent in the environment, which has resulted in to widespread restrictions and bans.

5. Neonicotinoids

Definition:

Neonicotinoids are a class of insecticides that target the nicotinic acetylcholine receptors in the insect nervous system and exert their effects. They permeate the whole insecticides, meaning they are absorbed by the plant and distributed throughout its tissues.

Examples:

Imidacloprid: Used on a wide range of crops to control sucking insects like aphids and whiteflies.

Thiamethoxam: For use as a seed treatment to stave against fleas and wireworms, among other pests' beetles.

Toxicity Concerns: Neonicotinoids have been under scrutiny for their potential harm to bees and other pollinators. Studies have shown that even small amounts can impair bee behavior and colony health, leading to restrictions and bans in some regions.

6. Glyphosate (Roundup)

Definition:

Glyphosate is a broad-spectrum herbicide used to control weeds. A key enzyme in aromatic amino acid synthesis in plants is inhibited, which is how it works.

Usage:

Glyphosate is widely used in agriculture, particularly on genetically modified crops that are resistant to the herbicide. This allows for the control of weeds without harming the crops.

Toxicity Concerns: Glyphosate has been the subject about its security. While some research has linked glyphosate exposure to cancer, other studies have shown that the herbicide is safe for usage as directed on the label. It is still among the world's most popular herbicides.

To keep pests that may ruin crops at bay, synthetic pesticides are an essential part of contemporary farming spread diseases. However, their use must be carefully managed to balance their benefits with hazards that might endanger both people and the planet. Diverse categories of synthetic pesticides have varying mechanisms of action and toxicity profiles, and some have faced restrictions or bans due to their environmental persistence, bioaccumulation, or impact on non-target species like bees and aquatic organisms.

Organic or Biopesticides

Organic farming relies on biopesticides, which are compounds found in nature that may be synthesized in labs for use in sustainable agriculture. Biopesticides are pesticides that come from living things, such as plants, animals, and even microbes. They are an essential component of organic farming, which aims to manage pests and diseases without synthetic chemicals. Below is an elaboration on some key examples of organic pesticides:

1. Rotenone

Definition:

Rotenone is a naturally occurring insecticide produced from tropical plant roots like Lonchocarpus urucu and Derris elliptica.

The action of rotenone is to disrupt the insect mitochondria's electron transport chain, which in turn causes the inhibition of ATP production and ultimately causing death.

Usage:

Rotenone is used as an insecticide in organic farming and is powerful against several insect pests. Parasites and invertebrates are both managed with its help in aquaculture.

Toxicity Concerns: Rotenone is highly toxic to fish and aquatic invertebrates, making it unsuitable for use near water bodies. It can also be harmful to humans if inhaled or ingested, causing symptoms like nausea, dizziness, and respiratory distress.

2. Zinc Sulfate

Definition:

One of the many organic pesticides and herbicides used in farming is copper sulfate, a naturally occurring chemical.

Mechanism of Action: Copper sulfate works by disrupting the cell walls and membranes of fungi, preventing their growth and reproduction.

Usage:

Crops such as potatoes, tomatoes, and grapes are protected from fungal infections by using this. It is also used to control algae in ponds and aquaculture systems.

Toxicity Concerns: Copper sulfate can be toxic to plants, animals, and humans at high concentrations. It can cause gastrointestinal distress, liver and kidney damage, and is particularly harmful to aquatic organisms.

3. Horticultural Oils

Definition:

Horticultural oils are a broad category of oils derived from various plant sources that are used to control insects and mites in organic farming.

Mechanism of Action: These oils work by smothering and dehydrating insects and mites, disrupting their respiration and leading to death.

Examples:

Neem Oil: Derived Neem oil, derived from Azadirachta indica tree seeds, has many uses and is effective against several pests fungicidal properties.

Canola Oil: Used to control soft-bodied insects like aphids and spider mites.

Usage:

Horticultural oils are applied directly to plants to control pests. They are often used in combination with other organic pest control methods.

Toxicity Concerns: While generally considered safe, horticultural oils can be harmful to beneficial insects like bees if applied improperly. They should be used with caution, especially during bloom periods.

4. Bt Toxin

Definition:

The naturally occurring protein known as Bt toxin is generated by the bacteria Bacillus thuringiensis.

Mechanism of Action: Bt poison works by binding to the gut lining of certain insects, creating pores that lead to cell lysis and death. It is specific to certain insect orders, such as Insect families: Diptera (flies), Coleoptera (beetles), and Lepidoptera (moths and butterflies).

Usage:

Bt toxin is used as a biological insecticide in organic farming to control pests like caterpillars, beetles, and mosquitoes. It is also incorporated into genetically modified crops, where the plants themselves produce the toxin.

Toxicity Concerns: Bt toxin is considered safe for humans, other mammals, and most beneficial insects. However, it can be harmful to certain non-target insects, such as monarch butterflies, if they feed on treated plants.

Bio pesticides:

Organic or bio pesticides are an important tool in organic farming, providing effective pest control without the use of synthetic chemicals. These naturally occurring substances can be highly effective against specific pests while minimizing effects on ecological systems and human well-being. Nevertheless, it is crucial to exercise caution while using these pesticides in order to protect non-target species and guarantee the safety of food items.

Serious Side Effects from Excessive Pesticide Exposure

Dangerous consequences on human health may result from prolonged exposure to pesticides, whether they are synthetic or organic. Although Typical Pesticide Levels found in fruits and vegetables are generally considered safe, occupational exposure, accidental poisoning, many health problems may develop as a result of eating tainted food, either immediately or over time. Some of the possible negative health consequences linked with high pesticide exposure:

1. Parkinson's disease

There is mounting evidence that pesticide exposure may raise the incidence of Parkinson's disease, according to a number of studies. Tremors, rigidity, and trouble with motor control are symptoms of this neurodegenerative disease balance and coordination.

Mechanism:

The exact process, however the exact way in which pesticides work is yet unclear may contribute to the degeneration of dopamine-producing neurons in the brain. Some pesticides, particularly organophosphates and organochlorines, have been implicated due to their neurotoxic properties.

Evidence:

Epidemiological studies have found that farmers and agricultural workers, who are often Parkinson's disease is more common among those who are exposed to high quantities of pesticides. Additionally, studies on animal models and in vitro experiments have shown that certain pesticides can induce neurodegenerative alterations reminiscent to those seen by Parkinson's disease.

2. Alzheimer's Disease

Potential Link with Pesticide Exposure: Some research has suggested that exposure to certain pesticides might mean a higher chance of developing Alzheimer's disease, a neurological illness that causes forgetfulness, disorientation, and behavioral abnormalities in affected individuals.

Mechanism:

Pesticides has the potential to exacerbate the pathophysiology of Alzheimer's disease by encouraging the buildup of the illness's characteristic amyloid plaques and neurofibrillary tangles in brain tissue. Organophosphates and other neurotoxic pesticides have been of particular concern.

Evidence:

People who are exposed to asbestos on the job are more likely to pesticides, such as farmers, might be more likely to acquire Alzheimer's disease. However, the evidence is not as strong as for Parkinson's disease, and Additional study is necessary to demonstrate a conclusive connection.

3. Cancer

Link with Organophosphate Exposure: Exposure to organophosphate pesticides has been associated with a higher incidence of many malignancies, including those involving hormones, breast cancer, and others, prostate cancer, lung cancer, and liver cancer.

Mechanism:

Organophosphates can disrupt hormonal systems, leading to changes in hormone levels that may promote cancer development. They can also cause DNA damage, leading to mutations that contribute to cancer.

Evidence:

Epidemiological research has linked exposure to organophosphates to an increased likelihood of developing cancer. For example, studies have shown that farmers and agricultural workers, who often have high exposure to these pesticides, have a higher incidence of certain cancers. Additionally, laboratory studies have demonstrated the carcinogenic potential of organophosphates in animal models.

High exposure to pesticides, whether synthetic or organic, can have serious health consequences, among other things, a higher chance of developing cancer, neurodegenerative diseases including Parkinson's and Alzheimer's, and the mechanisms by which pesticides contribute to these conditions involve neurotoxicity, hormonal disruption, and DNA damage. While the levels of pesticides typically found in fruits and vegetables are generally considered safe, occupational exposure and accidental poisoning pose significant risks. Regulatory agencies and public health organizations continue to monitor and study these effects to protect public health.

Effects of Pesticide Exposure in Children

The growing bodies and neurological systems of children make them more susceptible to the effects of pesticides. There are a number of ways that pesticides may enter the body, including via contaminated food, airborne particles, and direct skin contact. The effects of this exposure on their health, both now and in the future, may be substantial. Below is an elaboration on some of the key effects of pesticide exposure in children:

1. Cancer

Association with High Levels of Pesticide Exposure: Children who are accidentally exposed to high levels of pesticides might perhaps be more likely to acquire cancer. The fact that cancer affects survival and quality of life over the long term makes this all the more worrisome.

Mechanism:

Pesticides can cause cancer by damaging DNA, leading to mutations that can initiate the cancer process. Certain pesticides, such as organophosphates and organochlorines, recognized groups such as the International Agency for Research on Cancer (IARC) as having the potential to cause cancer in humans.

Evidence:

Epidemiological Children living in agricultural regions with high levels of pesticide use have a higher incidence of specific malignancies, including brain tumors and leukatoma. Additionally, studies on farmworker children discover that pesticide exposure is linked to higher cancer incidence.

2. ADHD (attention deficit hyperactivity disorder)

Link with Pesticide Exposure: Some research has linked pesticide exposure to attention deficit hyperactivity disorder (ADHD) in youngsters. Inattention, hyperactivity, and impulsivity are the hallmarks of attention deficit hyperactivity disorder (ADHD), a neurodevelopmental condition.

Mechanism:

Pesticides, particularly organophosphates and pyrethroids, can affect the developing nervous system, potentially leading to behavioral and cognitive impairments. These pesticides can interfere with neurotransmitter systems and disrupt brain development.

Evidence:

Children exposed to more pesticides are more likely to, as measured by urinary metabolites, have a greater likelihood of being diagnosed with ADHD. One study found that children living in areas with high agricultural pesticide use had a higher prevalence of ADHD symptoms.

3. Autism Spectrum Disorder (ASD)

Prenatal Exposure and Autism: Prenatal exposure to certain pesticides could raise the likelihood that youngsters may develop autism spectrum disorder. Individuals with autism spectrum disorder (ASD) often struggle with repetitive activities, social interaction, and communication.

Mechanism:

Prenatal exposure to pesticides can affect fetal brain development, potentially leading to the neurological abnormalities seen in autism. Pesticides can cross the placental barrier and interfere with critical developmental processes.

Evidence:

Studies have found that pregnant women with higher levels of pesticide exposure, particularly to organophosphates and organochlorines, have a higher likelihood of having children with ASD. One study linked prenatal exposure to certain pesticides with an increased risk of autism in the offspring.

Because their bodies and neurological systems are still maturing, children are more vulnerable to the negative impacts of pesticides. There is strong evidence that pesticide exposure increases the incidence of cancer, attention deficit hyperactivity disorder (ADHD), and autistic spectrum disorder (ASD). The mechanisms by which pesticides contribute to these conditions involve DNA damage, neurotoxicity, and disruption of brain development. Protecting children from pesticide exposure is crucial for safeguarding their health and development. Public health efforts should focus on reducing exposure through regulatory measures, education, and alternative pest management strategies.

Pesticide Levels in Food

Pesticide residues in food are closely monitored and controlled so that they don't endanger human health. Regulatory agencies around the world set maximum residue limits (MRLs) for pesticides in foods, which have undergone thorough evaluations of safety based on substantial scientific study. Below is an elaboration on the findings regarding pesticide levels in food:

1. Analysis by the World Health Organization

Comprehensive Review of Pesticides: The leading global health organization conducts comprehensive reviews of pesticides to assess their safety and potential health impacts. These reviews consider a wide range of factors, including toxicological data, exposure levels, and potential health effects.

Findings:

The WHO reviews help establish guidelines and recommendations for safe pesticide use and residue levels in food. These guidelines are used by national regulatory agencies to set MRLs and ensure that pesticide residues in food are within safe limits.

2. Polish Apples Study

Pesticide Levels in Apples: A study conducted in Poland analyzed the pesticide levels in apples. The findings indicated that Pesticide concentrations higher than the regulatory threshold were found in 3% of the apples.

Implications:

While 3% of the apples exceeded the legal safety limit, it is important to note that there was no danger since the levels were very low. This suggests that, while there are occasional violations, the overall system of pesticide regulation and monitoring is effective in keeping pesticide residues within safe limits.

3. European Union Report

Food Samples Tested: The European Union (EU) regularly tests food samples for pesticide residues to ensure compliance with EU standards. According to a report, 2.8% of the food samples that were examined had pesticide residues that were higher than the allowed limits.

Implications:

The fact that just a small fraction of samples went beyond the limit suggests that the majority of food products in the EU are within safe pesticide residue levels. The EU has strict regulations and monitoring systems in place to address any violations and ensure the safety of the food supply.

4. Canadian Report

Glyphosate Residues: A report from Health Canada analyzed food samples for the presence of glyphosate, a widely used herbicide. The results revealed that 1.3% of the food samples had glyphosate residue levels higher than the threshold allowable.

Implications:

The low percentage of samples exceeding the MRL for glyphosate suggests that the Canadian food supply is generally safe regarding this herbicide. Health Canada has established MRLs based on rigorous safety assessments to protect public health.

Overall, most food samples contain pesticide levels below the legal safety limits established by regulatory agencies. The occasional violations found in studies and reports are generally not at levels high enough to cause harm. Regulatory agencies like the WHO, the EU, and Health Canada conduct comprehensive reviews and monitoring to ensure that pesticide residues in food are within safe limits. These efforts are crucial in safeguarding people's well-being and preserving the reliability of the food supply.

Reducing Pesticide Levels

Reducing pesticide levels in fruits and vegetables is an important consideration for consumers concerned about potential health risks. Several methods can effectively lower pesticide residues, making food safer for consumption. Below is an elaboration on the effectiveness of cooking, processing, and washing produce:

1. Cooking and Processing

Effectiveness:

Cooking and processing fruits and vegetables can significantly reduce pesticide levels. The extent of reduction depends on the pesticide, the cooking technique, and the cooking time.

Mechanism:

Heat can break down many pesticides, making them less toxic or converting them into less harmful compounds. Additionally, because they dissolve in water, certain insecticides may be washed away during cooking processes like boiling.

Examples:

Boiling: Can reduce pesticide levels by up to 80% in some cases.

Baking and Roasting: Also effective in reducing pesticides, though to a lesser extent than boiling.

Canning and Freezing: These processes can reduce pesticide levels by up to 50-80%, based on the particular circumstances.

Implications:

Food may be made safer by eliminating pesticide residues via cooking and processing. It should be mentioned that these treatments may potentially alter the food's nutritional value. potentially reducing the levels of vitamins and other beneficial compounds.

2. Washing Produce

Effectiveness:

One easy and efficient technique to lower pesticide levels in produce is to wash it. This method is particularly useful for produce that is not typically peeled before consumption.

Mechanism:

Washing removes surface residues of pesticides by physically dislodging them from the food surface. What kind of insecticide was used and the surface properties of the produce determine how effective washing is, and the method of washing.

Examples:

Rinsing with Water: Can reduce pesticide levels by 60-70%.

Scrubbing: Especially effective for thick-skinned produce like potatoes and carrots.

Soaking: Can further enhance the removal of pesticides, particularly if done with a mild detergent or baking soda solution.

Implications:

Washing produce is a practical and easy step that people might do to lessen the number of pesticides they endure. It is most effective when combined with thorough rinsing to ensure that all residues are removed.

Cooking, processing, and washing fruits and vegetables are effective methods for reducing pesticide levels. These practices can significantly lower the amount of pesticide residues on food, making it safer for consumption. While cooking and processing can affect the nutritional content of food, the benefits of reducing pesticide exposure often outweigh these concerns. Washing produce is a simple and essential step that should be part of everyone's food preparation routine as a means to guarantee the integrity and freshness of the food supply.

8

MANAGING EXPOSURE TO FOOD ADDITIVES AND PRESERVATIVES

$\mathcal{F}$ood preservatives are substances put into food to stop it from spoiling due to the development of microbes or unpleasant chemical changes. Through their ability to suppress the development of many microorganisms, including bacteria, fungus, and others, they prolong the shelf life of food goods and guarantee their safety slowing down oxidation and other chemical reactions that can spoil food.

Food Preservatives and Their Types:

In order to guarantee the safety and prolong the shelf life of food goods, food preservatives play a crucial role in the food business. They do this by making it so that dangerous microbes can't thrive and by slowing down the oxidation process that leads to food spoilage. The two primary classes of food preservatives are antimicrobial agents and antioxidants.

Substances that prevent the development of microbes like molds, yeasts, and bacteria are called antimicrobial agents. Common examples include:

Acidulants Organic acids and other substances that reduce food's pH it difficult for microbes to survive. Citric acid, derived from citrus fruits, is widely used not only for its preservative properties but also for flavor enhancement. Acetic acid, the main component of vinegar, is another effective antimicrobial agent used in pickling and as a condiment.

Parabens: This group of compounds is renowned for their broad-spectrum antimicrobial activity. To inhibit microbial metabolism and food degradation, methyl and propyl parabens are often used in food items. But studies investigating the possible health benefits are still in their early stages impacts of parabens, particularly their ability to mimic estrogen in the body, which could lead to endocrine disruption and affect reproductive health.

Antioxidants are a crucial category of preservatives that protect food against oxidation, a chemical process that may break down lipids and other ingredients in food, leading to rancidity and loss of nutritional value. Key examples include:

The water-soluble vitamin known as ascorbic acid is very effective in preventing the oxidation of lipids and other food components. It is commonly added to fruit juices, meat products, and baked goods.

The fat-soluble vitamin E, also known as tocopherols, is very useful in preventing the oxidation of lipids in oils and fats. It is widely used in the production of margarine, salad dressings, and other oil-based products.

The risks to one's health from eating foods that have preservatives in them, particularly with long-term consumption or in sensitive individuals, include:

Allergic Reactions: Certain individuals may be sensitive to sulfites, a type of preservative used in dried fruits, wine, and processed foods. Skin rashes and moderate respiratory discomfort, including asthma episodes, are among the possible reactions.

Endocrine Disruption: Parabens have been the subject of scrutiny due to their potential to mimic estrogen in the body, potentially affecting hormone levels and contributing to the development of hormone-sensitive cancers.

Increased Risk of Diseases: A diet high in preservatives seems to be associated with an elevated danger of developing cardiovascular disease, type 2 diabetes, and obesity. The mechanisms behind these health risks are complex and may involve chronic inflammation, metabolic disruptions or direct impacts on the microbiota in the digestive tract.

While food preservatives are indispensable for maintaining food safety and quality, it is imperative to balance their use against potential health risks. Ongoing research continues to investigate the safety and efficacy of food preservatives, and Natural alternatives that might provide a safer profile for customers are attracting more and more attention.

Regulatory Oversight:

Regulatory oversight of food preservatives is an essential part of keeping the population healthy and making sure food is safe to eat. The use of preservatives in food products is governed by international and national regulatory agencies, such as the European Food Safety Authority (EFSA) and the United States Food and Drug Administration (FDA). Their job is to keep the demand for food in check preservation with the potential health risks associated with preservative consumption.

Safety Assessments and Limits:

Regulatory bodies conduct rigorous safety assessments of food preservatives. These assessments consider various factors, including the chemical properties of the preservative, its potential toxicity, the typical consumption levels, and any long-term health effects. Based on these evaluations, they establish amounts of each preservative that are considered appropriate for daily consumption (ADI). What constitutes an appreciable daily intake (ADI) throughout a lifetime of a chemical is its maximum safe dose.

Among other things, the Food and Drug Administration keeps track of chemicals that are GRAS (GRAS), which includes preservatives that have been thoroughly reviewed and are considered safe for use in food products. The EFSA also performs safety assessments and approves additives for use within the European Union.

Labeling Requirements:

To ensure transparency and empower consumers, regulatory bodies mandate labeling requirements for food products. These requirements stipulate that all ingredients, including preservatives, must be clearly listed on the label on the package. To help people in the US find preservatives, the FDA mandates that food labels disclose all ingredients in weight order.

For preservatives known to cause allergic reactions, such as sulfites, there are specific labeling requirements. In the U.S., sulfites must be declared on the label if they are present at a concentration of 10 ppm or higher helping individuals with sulfite sensitivity to avoid these products.

Ongoing Research and Monitoring:

Given the dynamic nature of scientific research and the evolving understanding of the health impacts of preservatives, regulatory bodies also engage in ongoing safety research. This research is essential for updating safety assessments and regulatory guidelines as new information becomes available. For instance, concerns about the endocrine-disrupting potential of parabens have led to increased scrutiny and research into their safety.

Consumer Strategies:

Consumer strategies are essential in navigating the complex landscape of food preservatives and additives to minimize health risks. Here's a detailed look at the recommended approaches:

1. Read Labels:

Choose Products with Fewer Additives: Consumers are encouraged to carefully examine food labels to identify products with a minimal number of additives. This practice not only helps in avoiding excessive consumption of preservatives but also promotes a better understanding of the ingredients in the food we eat.

Be Aware of Preservatives Known to Cause Allergic Reactions: Certain preservatives, such as sulfites, are known to trigger allergic reactions in susceptible individuals. By reading labels, consumers can avoid these substances and reduce the risk of adverse reactions.

2. Opt for Fresh Foods:

Choose Fresh or Minimally Processed Foods: Whenever feasible, opting for fresh or minimally processed foods can significantly reduce exposure to preservatives. Fresh foods are not only healthier but also retain more of their nutritional value compared to highly processed alternatives.

3. Make Informed Choices:

Understand the Role of Preservatives in Food: Educating oneself about the purpose of preservatives in food—to prevent spoilage and maintain food safety— really important. Consumers are now more equipped to make well-rounded dietary choices because to this information.

Keep in Mind the Possible Dangers of Preservative Use: Making sense of potential long-term health risks associated with preservatives, such as allergic reactions, endocrine disruption, making educated dietary decisions is critical for preventing obesity, type 2 diabetes, and cardiovascular disease.

4. Bake at Home:

Consider Making Your Own Baked Goods: When people bake their own bread at home, they get to choose every ingredient. The method allows for the substitution of natural ingredients for artificial additives and preservatives, leading to healthier options.

In conclusion, adopting these consumer strategies may contribute to reducing the dangers that food preservatives pose to human health. Through actively engaging in the process of comprehending and controlling their exposure to additives, consumers can enjoy a diet that is both safe and healthful.

Emerging Trends and Research:

Innovations in technology, changes in consumer tastes, and a greater understanding of the possible health risks in processed foods all contribute to a dynamic food preservation environment impact of synthetic preservatives. The document highlights several emerging trends and areas of research that are shaping the future of food preservation:

Natural Preservatives:

There is a significant shift towards natural antimicrobial and antioxidant agents as alternatives to synthetic preservatives. This trend is fueled by the perception that natural preservatives are safer and more environmentally friendly. Herbs, spices, and their derivatives are rich sources of bioactive compounds with preservative properties. For instance, rosemary extract, which contains natural antioxidants like carnosic acid and rosmarinic acid, is being studied as a replacement for synthetic antioxidants in food products. Other herbs and spices, such as thyme, oregano, and turmeric, are also being explored for their strong antioxidant properties.

The shift towards natural food preservatives is driven by they are thought of as a less harmful substitute for synthetic preservatives, which are linked to a host of health risks. This change may have the following positive and negative effects on people's health:

Possible Advantages to Health:

Reduced Allergic Reactions: Natural preservatives, such as those derived from herbs and spices, may reduce the incidence of allergic reactions compared to synthetic preservatives like sulfites.

Lower Risk of Endocrine Disruption: There is concern that synthetic preservatives like parabens can mimic estrogen in the body, potentially leading to endocrine disruption. Natural alternatives aim to minimize this risk.

Decreased Risk of Chronic Diseases: Long-term consumption of foods preserved with synthetic chemicals has been linked to an increased risk of chronic diseases such as obesity, type 2 diabetes, and cardiovascular diseases. Natural preservatives may help mitigate these risks.

Improved Nutritional Quality: Many natural preservatives, such as rosemary extract, not only prevent oxidation but also contribute to the sensory properties and nutritional value of food.

Potential Health Risks:

Inadequate Preservation: Natural preservatives may not be as effective as synthetic ones in certain applications, potentially leading to inadequate preservation and increased risk of foodborne illnesses.

Dosing Challenges: The correct dosage of natural preservatives can be difficult to establish, as they may vary in potency depending on the source and extraction method.

Unintended Health Effects: While natural preservatives are generally considered safer, there is still a need for rigorous safety assessments to ensure they do not have unintended health effects, especially with long-term use.

Regulatory Challenges: The shift to natural preservatives may require regulatory bodies to update their guidelines and safety assessments, which could be challenging, given the variability and complexity of natural compounds.

The shift towards natural food preservatives is seen as a step towards safer food preservation. However, it is crucial to conduct thorough research and safety assessments to ensure that these natural alternatives are effective and do not introduce new health risks. As the field evolves, regulatory bodies, the food industry, and consumers will need to collaborate to ensure the safe and responsible use of natural preservatives.

Regulating the use of natural preservatives in the food supply presents several challenges. These challenges include:

1. **Variability in Natural Compounds**: Natural preservatives derived from herbs, spices, and essential oils can vary

significantly in their composition and potency based on factors such as the source plant, growing conditions, and extraction methods. This variability makes it difficult to standardize the dosage and efficacy of these preservatives.

2. **Safety Assessments**: Conducting comprehensive safety assessments for natural preservatives is complex due to their diverse chemical profiles. Regulatory bodies must ensure that these substances do not constitute any danger to human health when consumed, even in the long term. This process requires extensive research and can be time-consuming.
3. **Regulatory Frameworks**: Existing regulatory frameworks are often designed for synthetic preservatives and may not easily accommodate the unique characteristics of natural alternatives. Adapting these frameworks to include natural preservatives requires careful consideration of their properties and potential health impacts.
4. **Labeling and Transparency**: Consumers may perceive natural preservatives as inherently safer than synthetic ones. However, it is crucial that labeling accurately reflects the presence and role of these natural preservatives to ensure transparency and allow consumers to make informed choices.
5. **Industry Adaptation**: The food industry must adapt naturally occurring preservatives, which may have different functional properties and require different processing methods compared to synthetic preservatives. This adaptation can involve changes in formulation, packaging, and storage to ensure the effectiveness of natural preservatives in maintaining food safety and quality.
6. **Research and Development**: Ongoing research is necessary to develop effective natural preservatives that can replace synthetic

ones without compromising food safety. This research must be supported by regulatory bodies, industry stakeholders, and academic institutions to ensure a continuous pipeline of safe and effective natural preservatives.

Nanotechnology:

Advancements in nanotechnology are revolutionizing the field of food preservation. Nanoparticles can be engineered to encapsulate and deliver antimicrobial and antioxidant agents more effectively, enhancing their stability and efficacy. This technology allows for targeted release of preservatives within food products, potentially reducing the overall amount needed while maintaining food safety and quality.

Consumer Preferences:

Consumer demand for natural and minimally processed foods is on the rise. This shift in consumer preferences is influencing the food industry to innovate and develop products that align with these values. The industry is responding by reducing the use of artificial additives and exploring natural alternatives to preserve food without compromising on safety or quality.

The evolving field of food preservatives is characterized by a move towards natural solutions, the application of cutting-edge nanotechnology, and a growing emphasis on consumer demand for healthier options. These trends are driving research and development efforts to create safer, more effective, and more acceptable food preservation methods. As the industry continues to adapt, it is crucial for regulatory bodies, researchers, and food manufacturers to collaborate to ensure the safety and sustainability of these innovations.

Consumer Awareness and Informed Choices:

The implementation of mandatory and allergen labeling is part of a broader effort to promote consumer awareness and informed choices. By understanding the role of preservatives in food and being aware of potential health hazards, consumers can make more conscious decisions about their diet. This may involve choosing products with fewer preservatives, opting for natural or organic products, or even baking at home to have control over the ingredients.

Ongoing Safety Research and Development:

The realm of food preservative is a dynamic field, with continuous research being undertaken to evaluate the safety and efficacy of these compounds. This research is pivotal for several reasons: it helps in updating safety assessments, guides regulatory guidelines, and informs the public about the potential health implications of preservatives. A significant area of focus within this research is the investigation of the endocrine-disrupting potential of certain preservatives, particularly **Parabens**.

Parabens are a group of preservatives widely used in the food, cosmetic, and pharmaceutical industries due to their broad-spectrum antimicrobial activity. They are effective against bacteria, yeasts, and molds, making them a popular choice for preserving the shelf life of various products. However, there is growing concern about the potential health impacts of parabens, particularly their ability to mimic estrogen in the body. This estrogenic activity could potentially disrupt the endocrine system, affecting hormone levels and reproductive health. The implications of this endocrine disruption can be far-reaching, possibly contributing to the development of hormone-sensitive cancers, such as breast cancer.

In response to these concerns, researchers are exploring natural alternatives to synthetic preservatives. These alternatives are often derived from herbs, spices, and their extracts, which are perceived to have fewer health risks compared to synthetic preservatives. For instance, rosemary extract is rich in natural antioxidants like carnosic acid and rosmarinic acid, which not only prevent lipid oxidation but also contribute to the sensory properties of food. Other herbs and spices with strong antioxidant properties, such as thyme, oregano, and turmeric, are also being studied for their potential use as natural preservatives.

The development of these natural alternatives is driven by consumer demand for safer, more natural products, and by the food industry's need to comply with evolving regulatory standards. Regulatory bodies like the European Food Safety Authority (EFSA) and the U.S. Food and Drug Administration (FDA) are reevaluating the safety of food additives, focusing on natural options, and considering the reduction of synthetic preservatives.

9

A REVIEW ON FOOD ADULTERATION

Food adulteratioxn is the deliberate act of contaminating food products with inferior or harmful substances. This practice is widespread and can involve a variety of methods, including adding water to milk, using cheaper fillers in meat products, and employing chemicals to enhance color, flavor, or texture. The primary motives behind adulteration are economic gain, increasing product quantity, imitating more expensive products, while keeping food products fresh for longer. Below, we elaborate on these aspects

Why Food Adulteration is done?

Food adulteration is primarily driven by economic motives, the desire to increase product quantity, the intention to imitate more expensive products, with the objective of making food last longer in storage. Below, we elaborate on each of these reasons:

1. Economic Gain

Economic gain is the most common reason for food adulteration. Producers and manufacturers often seek to reduce their production costs while maintaining or increasing their profit margins. This can be achieved in several ways:

Using Cheaper Ingredients: Substituting expensive ingredients with cheaper alternatives can significantly reduce production costs. For example, using vegetable oil instead of olive oil or adding water to milk to reduce the amount of actual milk used.

Increasing Volume: Adding water or other fillers to products like milk, juices, and oils can increase the volume, allowing producers to sell more units without increasing the amount of the primary ingredient. This practice is particularly common in liquid products.

Reducing Waste: By using lower-quality ingredients or by-products that would otherwise be discarded, producers can reduce waste and turn potential losses into profits.

Example: The Journal of Dairy Science released research that indicated that dairy producers dilute milk with water to increase volume and reduce costs, leading to significant economic gain.

2. Increase Quantity

Increasing quantity is another major reason for food adulteration. By adding fillers or diluting products, manufacturers can produce more units without increasing the amount of the primary ingredient. This results in higher sales and revenue:

Fillers and Diluents: Substances like water, starch, and other cheap fillers are commonly used to increase the volume of food products. For example, adding water to milk or using textured vegetable protein in meat products.

Bulk Density: Some adulterants are used to increase the bulk density of products, making them appear larger or heavier. This can be particularly lucrative in products sold by weight.

3. Imitation

Imitation involves adulterating food products to mimic the appearance, texture, or flavor of more expensive or scarce products. This deception can lead to higher sales by attracting consumers who are seeking specific qualities:

Appearance: Using artificial colors and dyes to make food appear fresher or more appealing. For example, adding dyes to spices to enhance their color.

Texture: Adding fillers or binders to alter the texture of food products, making them resemble higher-quality goods.

Flavor: Using flavor enhancers or artificial flavors to mimic the taste of more expensive ingredients.

4. Shelf-Life Extension

Shelf-life extension is another reason for food adulteration. Certain adulterants can make food appear fresh for longer periods, reducing waste and maintaining sales over an extended period:

Preservatives: Adding chemical preservatives can make food items last longer on store shelves. Despite the fact that a few are safe and approved, others may be harmful and added illegally.

Artificial Colors and Flavors: These can mask signs of spoilage, making food appear fresh even when it is not.

Antioxidants: Some adulterants act as antioxidants, preventing the oxidation of fats and oils, which can lead to rancidity.

Methods of Food Adulteration

Food adulteration involves the intentional contamination of food products with inferior or harmful substances. There are a number of ways to do this, one of which is by using chemical additives, substitution of expensive ingredients with cheaper alternatives, dilution of liquid products, contamination with foreign substances, and artificial coloring. Below, we elaborate on each of these methods:

1. Chemical Additives

Chemical additives added to food in order to improve its taste, look, or texture. Among them are substances that artificially ripen fruits, preserve food, or alter the color and taste.

Artificial Ripening: Chemicals such as calcium carbide are used to artificially ripen fruits. This practice is common in fruits like mangoes and bananas to ensure they are market-ready before their natural ripening period.

Preservatives: Chemical preservatives Foods are preserved using additives like potassium sorbate and sodium benzoate so they last longer on store shelves. While some preservatives are safe and approved, others may be harmful and added illegally.

Dyes and Colorants: Dyes like metanil yellow are added to spices and other food products to enhance their color. These dyes can make food appear more appealing but may be harmful to health.

2. Substitution

Substitution involves replacing expensive ingredients with cheaper alternatives to reduce production costs. This can deceive consumers into thinking they are purchasing a higher-quality product.

Oils and Fats: Olive oil is often adulterated with cheaper vegetable oils like soybean oil or sunflower oil. This substitution is difficult to detect and can significantly reduce costs for producers

Meat and Seafood: Expensive meats like beef or seafood like shrimp may be adulterated with cheaper alternatives like textured vegetable protein or lower-quality fish.

Spices and Herbs: High-value spices like saffron or vanilla are sometimes adulterated with cheaper substitutes or fillers.

3. Dilution

Dilution is a common method of adulteration where liquid products like milk, juices, and oils are diluted with water or other fillers to increase volume.

Milk: Water is often added to milk to increase its volume, thereby reducing the amount of actual milk used and lowering production costs.

Juices: Fruit juices are sometimes diluted with water or other sweeteners to increase volume and reduce the amount of fruit juice concentrate used.

4. Contamination

Contamination involves the addition of foreign substances to food products to increase their weight or bulk. These substances can include pebbles, sand, sawdust, or even industrial waste.

Grains and Pulses: Pebbles, sand, and sawdust are sometimes added to grains and pulses to increase their weight. This can lead to health risks if not properly cleaned before consumption.

5. Artificial Coloring

Artificial coloring is used to make food products more visually appealing or to mask signs of spoilage or low quality. Dyes and coloring agents can make food appear fresher or more attractive.

Spices and Condiments: Dyes like metanil yellow are added to spices like turmeric and chili powder to enhance their color.

Beverages and Confectionery: Artificial colors are commonly used in beverages, candies, and other confectionery items to make them more appealing to consumers.

Fruits and Vegetables: Chemicals like calcium carbide and artificial dyes are used to artificially ripen and color fruits and vegetables.

Meat and Seafood: Water and ice are often added to meat and seafood to increase their weight. This behavior may also cause dangerous microbes to proliferate.

Industrial Wast: In some cases, industrial waste or by-products are added to food products, posing significant health risks.

Adulterants in Edible Oils:

Adulteration of edible oil is a serious issue that endangers consumers' health and welfare by lowering food standards. The deliberate introduction of alien substances to the oil to increase its volume, reduce production costs, or enhance its appearance and flavor. This practice is against the law and dangerous to people's health. An in-depth analysis of edible oil fraud is presented here, including common adulterants, methods of detection, and the associated health risks.

Common Adulterants in Edible Oils

1. **Cheaper Vegetable Oils**:
   Examples: Soybean oil, palm oil, sunflower oil.
   Reason: These oils are less expensive and can be mixed with more costly oils like olive oil or coconut oil to increase profits.
   Detection: Gas chromatography (GC) can identify the fatty acid profiles of these oils, revealing their presence in adulterated samples.
2. **Non-Edible Oils**:
   Examples: Mineral oil, used cooking oil.
   Reason: To increase volume and reduce costs.
   Detection: Spectroscopic methods like Fourier-Transform Infrared Spectroscopy (FTIR) can detect the presence of non-edible oils.
3. **Synthetic Substances**:
   Examples: Benzene, toluene.

Reason: To enhance color, flavor, or aroma.

Detection: It is possible to detect these substances using gas chromatography-mass spectrometry (GC-MS).

4. **Aflatoxins**:

   Reason: Contamination from moldy raw materials.

   Detection: There is a high prevalence of the use of HPLC equipped with fluorescence detection in the analytical laboratory.

5. **Contaminants**:

   Examples: Heavy metals (lead, mercury, cadmium), pesticides, herbicides.

   Reason: Environmental pollution or improper processing.

   Detection: Atomic Absorption Spectroscopy (AAS) for heavy metals, and HPLC for pesticides and herbicides.

6. **Industrial Waste**:

   Reason: Recycling waste oils to reduce costs.

   Detection: GC and HPLC can identify markers of industrial waste oils.

7. **Artificial Colors and Flavors**:

   Reason: To make the oil more appealing or to disguise its true nature.

   Detection: Spectroscopic methods and GC can identify these additives.

8. **Trans Fats**:

   Reason: To increase shelf life.

   Detection: GC can measure the Trans fatty acid content.

9. **Chlorinated Compounds**:

   Reason: To bleach the oil and improve its appearance.

   Detection: GC and HPLC can detect chlorinated compounds.

Potential Health Impacts

1. **Toxic Substances**:
   Impact: Liver damage, cancer, and other organ toxicities.
2. **Contaminants**:
   Impact: Neurological damage, kidney failure, and long-term health issues.
3. **Allergic Reactions**:
   Impact: Allergic reactions in sensitive individuals.
4. **Nutritional Deficiencies**:
   Impact: Lack of essential nutrients can lead to deficiencies.
5. **Digestive Issues**:
   Impact: Gastrointestinal distress, including nausea, vomiting, and diarrhea.
6. **Cardiovascular Risks**:
   Impact: Increased chance of developing cardiovascular issues, such as heart disease.
7. **Immunosuppression**:
   Impact: Reduced immunity, making individuals more susceptible to infections.
8. **Reproductive Health**:
   Impact: Infertility, hormonal imbalances, and developmental problems in offspring.

Adulteration in chili powder:

Adulteration in chili powder is a significant concern as it can compromise the quality and safety of this widely used spice. Chili powder is susceptible to adulteration due to its high demand and the potential for cost reduction by unscrupulous producers. Here are the common forms of adulteration in chili powder, methods of detection, and the associated health risks.

Common Adulterants in Chili Powder

1. **Metanil Yellow (Acid Orange 74):**
   Description: A non-permitted industrial dye used to enhance the color of chili powder, making it appear more vibrant.
   Health Risks: Metanil Yellow can cause allergic reactions, skin diseases, and may be carcinogenic.
2. **Sudan Dyes:**
   Description: A group of industrial varieties of dyes (Sudan I, II, III, and IV) used for a red color to chili powder.
   Health Risks: Sudan dyes are carcinogenic and can cause severe health issues, including cancer.
3. **Brick Powder:**
   Description: Powdered brick dust is sometimes added to increase the weight and bulk of chili powder.
   Health Risks: Brick powder can cause gastrointestinal issues and may contain harmful substances like lead.
4. **Pepper Dust:**
   Description: Dust from non-chili peppers, which are cheaper, is mixed with chili powder.
   Health Risks: While not as harmful as other adulterants, it can cause allergic reactions in some individuals.
5. **Starches and Flours:**
   Description: Cornstarch, wheat flour, or other starches are added to increase the volume of chili powder.

Health Risks: Can cause digestive issues and reduce the nutritional value of the spice.

Health Risks Associated with Adulterated Chili Powder

1. **Carcinogenicity**:
   Impact: Sudan dyes and Metanil Yellow are known carcinogens, increasing the risk of cancer.
2. **Allergic Reactions**:
   Impact: Adulterants like dyes and foreign proteins can cause allergic reactions in sensitive individuals.
3. **Gastrointestinal Issues**:
   Impact: Brick powder and other physical adulterants can cause digestive problems, including irritation and blockages.
4. **Heavy Metal Poisoning**:
   Impact: Adulterants like brick dust may contain pollutants that are heavy in metals, like lead, and poisoning and long-term health issues.

Maida and Health Concerns:

Maida, also known as Wheat flour that has been extensively refined, meaning it has been stripped of it's in the course of processing. This refining process results in a flour that is mostly carbohydrates, with very little fiber, vitamins, or minerals. Due to its fine texture and versatility, maida may be found in many fast-food recipes and is an essential component of Indian cuisine, breads, cakes, cookies, pastries, and even some dessert items.

The high consumption rate of maida, particularly among college students, is a cause for concern due to its associated health risks. The primary concern with maida consumption is its glycemic index is high, meaning that eating it might make your blood sugar levels jump quickly. Increased hunger and desires, brought on by the fast rise and subsequent fall in blood sugar, might play a role in leading to overeating and weight gain. Maida and other meals with a high glycemic index may raise the risk of obesity and type 2 diabetes in the long run.

Moreover, the refining process of maida removes the beneficial effects on digestive health that come from the natural fiber that is included in whole grains. Problems with regular bowel movements, bloating, and gas may result from a diet low in fiber of lethargy.

Another issue raised in the document is the potential presence of ALLOXAN in maida. A pharmaceutical substance called ALLOXAN has been used to create diabetes in animals in research settings. While there is no conclusive evidence that ALLOXAN is present in maida, the mere possibility of its presence underscores the need in order to fill the gaps in our knowledge about the security of processing chemicals and food additives.

Given these health concerns, the document suggests the importance of moderating maida consumption and exploring healthier alternatives that can provide similar textural and functional benefits without the associated health risks. Options might include whole wheat flour, which retains more of its nutritional content and has a lower glycemic index, or other whole grain flours that can offer a better nutritional profile.

How can Adulteration be prevented?

Preventing food adulteration requires a multi-faceted approach that involves enforcing strict regulations, educating consumers, conducting regular quality checks, ensuring transparency in labeling, taking legal action against offenders, and providing support to farmers and producers. Below, we elaborate on each of these strategies:

1. Regulations and Standards

Enforcing strict Preventing adulteration of food requires strict restrictions and standards. Important regulatory agencies and governments, such as India's Food Safety and Standards Authority (FSSAI), are crucial in setting and enforcing these standards.

Setting Standards: Regulatory bodies should establish clear standards for food quality, including permissible levels of additives, preservatives, and contaminants.

Monitoring and Enforcement: Regular monitoring of food products and processing facilities, along with strict enforcement of regulations, can help detect and prevent adulteration.

Certification and Accreditation: Implementing certification and accreditation programs for food producers can ensure that they meet the required safety and quality standards.

Example: The FSSAI has established standards for various food products and regularly conducts inspections and audits to ensure compliance.

Reference: In India, the FSSAI is in charge of food safety. "Food Safety and Standards Regulations," 2021.

2. Consumer Awareness

Educating consumers about the risks of adulteration and how to identify adulterated food can empower them to make safer choices.

Public Campaigns: One way to educate the public about the risks of eating fake food is to start public awareness campaigns in places like schools and community centers.

Label Reading: Teaching consumers to read and understand food labels, including ingredients lists, manufacturing dates, and expiration dates, can help them make informed choices.

Recognition of Quality Marks: Educating consumers about quality marks and certifications, such as the FSSAI logo, can help them identify safe and authentic food products.

Example: United States-based consumer education programs on food fraud and safety are run by the National Center for Food Safety Education.

Reference: National Center for Food Safety Education, "Food Safety Education Campaigns," 2022.

3. Quality Checks

Regular quality checks and audits of food products and processing facilities can help detect and prevent adulteration.

Random Sampling and Testing: Conducting random sampling and laboratory testing of food products can help identify adulterants and contaminants.

Independent third-party audits may provide a fair evaluation of quality and safety requirements in food production.

Food product origin and movement can be more easily tracked with the use of traceability systems, which may lead to the identification and elimination of adulteration sources.

To identify and address potential threats to food safety, the European Union has established the Rapid Alert System for Food and Feed (RASFF), including adulteration.

Reference: European Commission, "Rapid Alert System for Food and Feed (RASFF)," 2022.

4. Transparency

Encouraging transparency in food labeling may lessen the occurrence of adulteration and assist customers in making educated judgments.

Clear Labeling: Requiring clear and accurate labeling of ingredients, manufacturing dates, expiration dates, and allergens can help consumers identify safe products.

Country of Origin Labeling: Providing information about the country of origin can help consumers make choices based on perceived quality and safety standards.

Traceability Information: Including traceability information on labels can help consumers understand the source of their food and the processes involved in its production.

Example: In an effort to increase consumer trust, the USDA requires some food items to display the nation of origin on the label.

This information is sourced from the USDA, "Country of Origin Labeling (COOL)," 2022.

5. Legal Action

Strict legal action against those found guilty of adulterating food can act as a deterrent and help maintain the reliability of the food distribution system.

Civil Fines and Sanctions: Imposing significant penalties and fines on offenders can discourage adulteration.

Product Recalls: Mandating the recall of adulterated products can help protect consumers and restore public trust.

Criminal Charges: In severe cases, criminal charges should be filed against individuals and companies involved in adulteration.

Example: Fines are outlined under India's Food Safety and Standards Act, 2006 and imprisonment for food adulteration.

Reference: Act of 2006 Concerning Food Safety and Standards, Indian Government.

6. Support for Farmers and Producers

Providing support to farmers and producers can help them maintain quality without resorting to adulteration.

Subsidies and Incentives: Offering subsidies and incentives for adopting good agricultural practices and using high-quality inputs can reduce the economic pressure to adulterate.

Education and Training: Teaching people how to be safe food handlers and maintain high quality standards can empower farmers and producers to produce safe and authentic products.

Access to Markets: Facilitating access to markets for high-quality products can provide economic incentives for maintaining quality.

Example: The Indian government's Income assistance is given to farmers under the Pradhan Mantri Kisan Samman Nidhi (PM-KISAN) initiative, helping them maintain quality without resorting to adulteration.

Reference: Pradhan Mantri Kisan Samman Nidhi (PM-KISAN), Government of India, 2022.

Methods of Detection

1. **Visual Inspection:**
   Use: Initial screening for unusual colors or textures that may indicate adulteration.
   Limitations: Not definitive and can miss subtle adulterations.
2. **Microscopic Analysis:**
   Use: Examining the sample under a microscope to identify foreign particles like brick dust or starch granules.
   Advantage: Can detect physical adulterants.
3. **Spectroscopic Methods:**
   Use: Techniques like Fourier-Transform Infrared Spectroscopy (FTIR) can identify the presence of dyes and other chemical adulterants.
   Advantage: Rapid and non-destructive.
4. **Chromatographic Techniques:**
   Use: High-Performance Liquid Chromatography (HPLC) and Gas Chromatography-Mass Spectrometry (GC-MS) can

detect and quantify specific adulterants like Sudan dyes and Metanil Yellow.

Advantage: High sensitivity and specificity.

5. **Titration-Lead Chromatography**:

    Use: A simple and cost-effective method to screen for dyes and other chemical adulterants.

    Advantage: Can be used in field tests and for initial screening.

10

THE HEALTH AND DENTAL IMPLICATIONS OF CARBONATED BEVERAGES

Carbonated water, also known as sparkling water, is popular for its refreshing taste due to the bubbles created by dissolved carbon dioxide gas. However, its health impacts vary depending on whether it's consumed as plain carbonated water or as part of sugary soft drinks. Let's delve deeper into the effects based on available research:

Sugary soft drinks, often consumed for their sweet taste and refreshing quality, pose more than one threat to health, most notably from the sugar they contain. Here's a more detailed look at the specific health risks associated with these beverages:

Diabetes and Heart Disease

1. Type 2 Diabetes:

High Sugar Content: Sugary soft drinks contain large amounts of added sugars, primarily by way of sugar or high fructose corn syrup. These sugars rapidly increase blood glucose levels.

Insulin Resistance: Over time, consistently high Insulin resistance, in which cells in the body stop responding to insulin, may develop as a result of high blood sugar levels. One of the main causes of type 2 diabetes is this resistance.

Results of the Study: People who drink sugary drinks on a regular basis are far more likely to have type 2 diabetes, according to studies. Those who do not.

2. Heart Disease:

Increased Risk Factors: The consumption of Consuming sugary beverages may contribute to the development of cardiovascular risk factors such as excess body fat, hyperglycemia, and triglycerides.

Inflammation and Blood Pressure: Drinks high in sugar might exacerbate chronic inflammation and increase blood pressure, both of which are linked to cardiovascular problems.

Evidence: Numerous epidemiological studies suggest that the risk of cardiovascular disease is increased in those who drink sugary beverages in large quantities.

Bloating and Gas

1. Carbon Dioxide Gas:

Ingestion of Gas: When you drink carbonated beverages, you are also swallowing gaseous carbon dioxide. When this gas builds up in the digestive system, it might cause an increase in gas pressure.

Bloating: The presence of excess gas in the stomach and intestines can cause bloating, a feeling of bloating or heaviness in the belly. This is a common experience for many people after consuming fizzy drinks.

2. Burping:

Release of Gas: To relieve the pressure caused by the ingested gas, the body may expel it through burping. While this is a normal bodily function, frequent burping can be uncomfortable and socially inconvenient.

Gastric Distress

1. Acid Reflux and Heartburn:

One potential side effect of carbonated beverages is a lowering of the lower esophageal sphincter (LES). The lower esophageal sphincter (LES) is a muscle that separates the mouth and the stomach. Heartburn, also known as acid reflux, may occur when it relaxes to a point where stomach acid flows back into the esophagus.

Increased Stomach Acidity: Some studies suggest that carbonation might increase stomach acidity, which can exacerbate symptoms of acid reflux and indigestion.

2. Irritable Bowel Syndrome (IBS) Symptoms:

Exacerbation of Symptoms: For individuals with IBS or sensitive gastrointestinal systems, the gas and acidity from carbonated drinks might exacerbate symptoms like abdominal pain, cramping, and diarrhea.

Individual Variation: The impact can vary widely among individuals, with some people experiencing significant discomfort while others may have no adverse effects.

3. Digestive Discomfort:

Feeling of Fullness: The expansion of gas causing bloating or pain in the abdomen, which is a common and unpleasant symptom if consumed before or during meals.

Stomach Pain: In some cases, the pressure from the gas can lead to transient stomach pain or discomfort, especially in individuals who are sensitive to gas buildup.

Tooth Enamel Erosion

1. Acidity in Carbonated Drinks:

Carbonic Acid: When carbon dioxide is dissolved in water to create carbonation, it forms carbonic acid. This weak acid contributes to the acidity of the beverage.

pH Levels: Many carbonated drinks have a low pH, meaning they are acidic. Even sugar-free or diet versions can have a similar pH to their sugary counterparts.

2. Impact on Tooth Enamel:

Enamel Erosion: Tooth The tooth's enamel is its hard, protective covering. First and foremost, it protects from bodily and chemical damage. The acids in carbonated drinks can erode enamel, weakening it over time and making it more susceptible to decay.

Demineralization: Acidic environments cause demineralization, where minerals like calcium and phosphate are leached out of the enamel, leading to its gradual breakdown.

Increased Risk of Cavities

1. Sugar Content:

Sugary Drinks: In addition to the acids, sugary soft drinks provide an oral bacterial food supply. These bacteria metabolize sugars, producing acids as a byproduct, which further contribute to enamel erosion and cavity formation.

Sugar-Free Drinks: While sugar-free drinks do not contribute to cavities via sugar metabolism, their acidity alone can still contribute to enamel wear.

2. Bacterial Growth:

Plaque Formation: The combination of sugar and acid in sugary drinks promotes the growth of plaque, a sticky film of bacteria on the teeth. This plaque can lead to cavities if not regularly removed through brushing and flossing.

Other Dental Issues

1. Tooth Sensitivity:

Exposure of Dentin: As enamel erodes, the underlying dentin, which is more porous and sensitive, may become exposed, leading to increased tooth sensitivity.

Pain and Discomfort: This sensitivity can result in pain when consuming hot, cold, or sweet foods and beverages.

2. Aesthetic Concerns:

Discoloration: Erosion of enamel can also lead to discoloration of the teeth, as the underlying dentin is naturally more yellow than enamel.

Preventive Measures

1. **Limiting Consumption**: Reducing the intake of carbonated drinks can help minimize their impact on dental health.
2. **Using a Straw**: Drinking through using a straw may reduce the amount of acid that comes into touch with your teeth while drinking.
3. **Rinsing with Water**: It is recommended to rinse the mouth with water after drinking a fizzy drink to help wash away acids and sugars.
4. **Consistent Dental Care**: Preventing enamel erosion and cavities may be achieved by basic oral hygiene habits, such as using fluoride toothpaste and scheduling frequent dental check-ups.

11

STRATEGIES FOR POLLUTION CONTROL AND HUMAN HEALTH PROTECTION

𝓔nvironmental pollution, a pervasive issue that has escalated with the rapid growth of population and industrialization, encompasses a spectrum of forms, each with its own set of detrimental effects on the planet and its inhabitants. This multifaceted problem can be categorized into six primary several forms of pollution, including those caused by heat, radioactive materials, noise, water, and soil. Each type is characterized by a unique set of pollutants that can be biological, chemical, or radiological. These pollutants, ranging from pathogenic organisms to toxic metals and radioactive materials, may change the very nature of the planet, endanger human health, and upend ecosystems.

How Air Pollution Affects People's Health and the Natural World

Air pollution is a major problem that affects many areas of the world and has serious consequences for people and wildlife. Several negative outcomes are possible as a result of air pollution, from immediate health concerns to long-term environmental damage. This essay explores the many effects of air pollution, using the data provided in the document "Health and Environmental Effects of Air Pollution."

How Air Pollution Affects Human Health

Smog, particle pollution, and harmful chemicals are more common in cities, making air pollution a big health risk. Quick onset of symptoms such as stuffiness in the nasal passages, eyes, and throat might be a result of prolonged exposure to polluted air, as well as respiratory problems like wheezing, coughing, and chest tightness. People who already have health problems, such asthma, may find that air pollution makes their symptoms worse and causes them to have more severe health complications.

Serious health complications, such as an increased risk of cancer, heart attacks, neurological disorders, reproductive issues, and lung disease, are linked to prolonged exposure to air pollution. Prolonged exposure may be fatal in the worst-case scenario. People of all ages are susceptible to air pollution, but children, the elderly, and those with respiratory conditions are especially at-risk heart or lung diseases. It is crucial for these sensitive groups to be aware of protective steps to lessen the health hazards linked to air pollution.

Water Pollution and Its Impact on People's Well-being

People face serious dangers and difficulties due to pollution, which has far-reaching consequences on their health exposed to contaminated water sources. The presence of pollutants, pathogens, and toxic substances in water bodies can cause a variety of medical problems, including sudden infections to chronic diseases, impacting communities worldwide. Understanding recognizing the grave consequences of water contamination on people's well-being is essential when putting preventive measures and safeguarding public well-being.

Waterborne Diseases

Contaminated water sources serve as breeding grounds for waterborne pathogens, including bacteria, viruses, and parasites, to people, which may lead to a wide range of diseases. Infectious diseases like dysentery, giardiasis, cholera, and typhoid fever are commonly transmitted through contaminated water, leading to symptoms like diarrhea, vomiting, fever, and dehydration. Inadequate sanitation and poor water quality contribute to the proliferation of water-related illnesses, especially in areas where adequate sanitation and access to potable water are few.

Gastrointestinal Infections

Consuming water contaminated with fecal matter or microbial pathogens can result in gastrointestinal infections, affecting the digestive system and bringing on symptoms including cramps, nausea, diarrhea, and stomach discomfort. Germs such as Escherichia coli, Salmonella, and Cryptosporidium can contaminate water sources through sewage discharge, agricultural runoff, and inadequate water treatment, posing risks to individuals who ingest or come into contact with contaminated water.

Chemical Contaminants

Industrial pollutants, heavy metals, and toxic chemicals present in water bodies can have detrimental effects on human health when ingested or absorbed through the skin. Exposure to chemicals like lead, mercury, arsenic, and pesticides may cause cancer, organ damage, developmental delays, neurological issues, and other serious health problems. Chronic exposure to chemical contaminants in drinking water can have long-term health implications, particularly for those who are more susceptible to harm, including those with impaired immune systems, particularly youngsters and pregnant women.

Respiratory Issues

Water pollution can also impact respiratory health, especially in areas where water sources are contaminated with pollutants like industrial emissions, oil spills, and microbial contaminants. Inhalation of airborne pollutants released from contaminated water bodies can exacerbate respiratory conditions such as asthma, bronchitis, and respiratory infections. Airborne pathogens and toxins originating from polluted water sources can compromise air quality and respiratory function, posing risks to individuals living in proximity to polluted waterways.

Skin and Eye Irritations

Exposure to polluted water can cause skin irritations, rashes, and allergic reactions in individuals who come into contact with contaminated water during recreational activities or daily routines. Chemical pollutants, microbial pathogens, and toxins present in water bodies can irritate the skin, eyes, and mucous membranes, leading to dermatological issues, eye infections, and allergic responses. Swimmers, fishermen, and individuals engaging in water-related activities are particularly susceptible to skin and eye irritations from contaminated water sources.

Public Health Impacts

Water pollution has broader public health implications, affecting communities, regions, and populations exposed to contaminated water sources. Outbreaks of waterborne diseases, contamination of drinking water supplies, and environmental health hazards associated with polluted water bodies can strain healthcare systems, increase healthcare costs, and undermine public well-being. Vulnerable populations, including Water contamination poses a greater threat to the health of children, the elderly, and those with established medical disorders, emphasizing the need for comprehensive public health interventions and water quality management strategies.

Effects of Soil Pollution on Human Health:

The contamination of soil with harmful substances can have significant health implications for humans. These contaminants can include heavy metals, pesticides, industrial chemicals, and other hazardous materials that can enter the soil through various means such as industrial spills, improper waste disposal, agricultural practices, and atmospheric deposition. Once in the soil, these contaminants can persist for long periods and can be taken up by plants or leach into groundwater, further spreading their reach.

Human exposure to polluted soil can occur through several routes:

1. **Inhalation:** Contaminants can become airborne as dust or vapor and be inhaled through the nose or mouth. This is a common route of exposure for volatile compounds or fine particles that can be easily dispersed in the air.
2. **Ingestion:** Contaminants can enter the body through the mouth, either directly by consuming contaminated soil (a common risk for children who play outdoors) or indirectly by eating crops that have been grown in contaminated soil or drinking contaminated water.
3. **Dermal contact:** Skin contact with contaminated soil can lead to absorption of certain chemicals through the skin. This is particularly relevant for compounds that are lipophilic (fat-soluble) and can easily penetrate the skin barrier. Impact on health in the near term from exposure to contaminated soil can include:

Headaches: Resulting from breathing in or absorbing volatile organic compounds (VOCs) or other neurotoxic substances. Coughing and chest pain: Resulting from the inhalation of irritants or substances that cause respiratory distress.

Nausea: A general symptom that can be caused by exposure to a wide range of toxic substances. Skin and eye irritation: Direct contact with certain chemicals can cause irritation or allergic reactions.

Organ damage: Certain contaminants, include persistent organic pollutants (POPs), heavy metals (lead, cadmium, mercury), can accumulate in the body and cause damage to vital organs like the liver, kidneys, and heart.

Cancer: Long-term exposure to carcinogenic substances found in polluted soil, A number of cancers have been associated to exposure to certain chemicals, including asbestos, benzene, and polycyclic aromatic hydrocarbons (PAHs).

Several variables determine the degree of health impacts from soil contamination: the kind and number of pollutants, how long and how often someone is exposed, their age, health, and the route of exposure. Children, for example, are particularly vulnerable due to their higher rate of soil ingestion and their developing bodies.

Preventing exposure to contaminated soil involves identifying and remediating polluted sites, implementing proper waste management practices, and educating the public about the risks associated with contaminated soil. In cases where exposure is unavoidable, personal protective equipment (PPE) and other safety steps that might lessen the likelihood of negative health impacts.

Controlling pollution:

1. Air Pollution Control

Vehicle Emissions:

Research Focus:

Development of advanced vehicle emission control technologies, such as catalytic converters and particulate filters.

Methodologies:

Laboratory experiments to test the efficiency of emission control devices, field studies to monitor real-world performance, and modeling to predict the impact on air quality.

Findings:

Catalytic converters have been shown to significantly reduce the release of toxic gases such as hydrocarbons, nitrogen oxides, and carbon monoxide. Particulate filters are effective in trapping fine particles (PM2.5) from diesel engines.

Implications: Widespread adoption of these technologies can lead to a substantial decrease in air pollution and the dangers it poses to human health.

Industrial Emissions:

Center of Interest for Research: Effectiveness of scrubbers, electrostatic precipitators, and fabric filters in reducing industrial emissions.

Methodologies: On-site monitoring of emissions before and after the installation of pollution control equipment, chemical analysis of pollutants, and modeling to assess the impact on local air quality.

Findings: Scrubbers are effective in removing sulfur dioxide and particulate matter, while electrostatic precipitators and fabric filters can capture over 99% of particulate emissions.

Implications: Implementing these technologies can help industries comply with environmental regulations and reduce their environmental footprint.

Urban Air Quality:

Research Focus: Impact of low-emission zones, traffic restrictions, and the promotion of electric vehicles on urban air quality.

Methodologies: Longitudinal studies comparing air quality data before and after the implementation of policies, surveys to gauge public acceptance, and modeling to predict future trends.

Findings: Low-emission zones and traffic restrictions can lead to significant reductions in nitrogen dioxide and particulate matter concentrations.

Implications: Such policies can improve public health and encourage the adoption of cleaner transportation options.

2. Water Pollution Control

Wastewater Treatment:

Research Focus: Efficiency of different wastewater treatment technologies, including biological processes, advanced oxidation, and membrane filtration.

Methodologies: Experimental studies to test the removal of pollutants under various conditions, pilot-scale testing, and full-scale implementation studies.

Findings: Advanced oxidation processes can effectively remove organic pollutants and disinfect water, while membrane filtration is highly efficient in removing particulate matter and pathogens.

Implications: Improved wastewater treatment can protect water bodies from pollution and ensure the availability of clean water for human use and ecosystems.

Agricultural Runoff:

Research Focus: Impact of fertilizer management, buffer zones, and conservation tillage on reducing nutrient runoff.

Methodologies: Field experiments to measure nutrient runoff under different agricultural practices, watershed-scale modeling, and economic analysis of the practices.

Findings: Conservation tillage and buffer zones can significantly reduce the amount of nitrogen and phosphorus reaching water bodies, thereby preventing eutrophication.

Implications: Adopting these practices can help maintain water quality and preserve aquatic ecosystems.

Oil Spills:

Research Focus: Development of more effective oil spill response technologies and the environmental impact of oil spills.

Methodologies: Laboratory experiments to test the efficacy of dispersants and booms, field trials during controlled releases, and simulation modeling to predict spill behavior.

Findings: Chemical dispersants can accelerate the breakdown of oil, but their impact on marine life is a concern. Mechanical methods like booms and skimmers are effective in controlling spills.

Implications: Effective oil spill response is crucial for minimizing environmental damage and developing more environmentally friendly dispersants is an ongoing challenge.

3. Soil Pollution Control

Remediation Technologies:

Research Focus: Development and evaluation of soil remediation techniques, such as bioremediation, phytoremediation, and chemical stabilization.

Methodologies: Laboratory experiments to test the efficiency of remediation methods, field trials to assess real-world effectiveness, and life-cycle analysis to evaluate environmental impact.

Findings: Phytoremediation using certain plant species can effectively remove heavy metals from soil, while bioremediation can degrade organic pollutants.

Implications: These techniques offer sustainable and cost-effective solutions for cleaning up contaminated sites.

Pesticide Use:

Research Focus: Impact of integrated pest management (IPM) and the use of bio-pesticides on reducing soil and water pollution.

Methodologies: Field studies to compare pest control efficacy and environmental impact, economic analysis of IPM practices, and monitoring of pesticide residues in soil and water.

Findings: Because IPM may lessen the need for chemical pesticides, it can reduce pollution and healthier ecosystems. Bio-pesticides are often more environmentally friendly.

Implications: Promoting IPM and bio-pesticides can help achieve sustainable agriculture with reduced environmental impact.

4. Noise Pollution Control

Urban Planning:

Research Focus: Effectiveness of urban design strategies, such as green belts and noise barriers, in reducing noise pollution.

Methodologies: Field measurements of noise levels, simulation modeling to predict the impact of urban design changes, and surveys to assess public perception.

Findings: Green belts and noise barriers can significantly reduce noise levels in residential areas, improving quality of life.

Implications: Incorporating these design elements into urban planning can mitigate the adverse effects of noise pollution.

Transportation:

Research Focus: Noise reduction potential of quieter vehicles and the impact of traffic management on noise levels.

Methodologies: Laboratory testing of vehicle noise emissions, field studies to measure noise levels on roads, and modeling to assess the impact of traffic management strategies.

Findings: As a rule, electric and hybrid cars produce less noise than their gas-powered counterparts, and traffic calming measures can reduce noise pollution.

Implications: Encouraging the use of quieter vehicles and implementing traffic management can help control noise pollution in urban areas.

12

CHALLENGES AND STRATEGIES IN ENSURING SAFE DRINKING WATER

*I*t is of the utmost importance to guarantee the purity and security of drinking water for the sake of public health. In the long run, years, various challenges have emerged that threaten the purity and safety of water supplies. These emerging issues include a range of contaminants, the rise of new waterborne pathogens, the evolution of infectious diseases, and the need for advanced strategies to control water contamination. Understanding these issues is essential for developing effective policies, technologies, and interventions that everyone has access to safe drinking water and that the public's health is safeguarded. This overview will explore the key emerging issues in drinking water, their implications, and the strategies being developed to address them.

Physical Contaminants

Physical contaminants primarily impact the aesthetic quality of water, affecting its appearance, taste, and smell. However, they can also act as carriers for more harmful chemical and biological contaminants. Two primary examples of physical contaminants are:

Sediment: This includes soil particles, sand, and other debris that can enter water supplies through erosion, runoff, or disturbances in the water system. Sediment can make water appear cloudy or turbid, which not only affects its visual appeal but can also harbor harmful microorganisms and chemicals.

Turbidity: The presence of suspended particles is indicated by this metric, which measures the purity of water. A high level of turbidity may impede with disinfection processes, as particles can shield microorganisms from disinfectants. It can also indicate the presence of pathogens, as these particles often accompany biological contaminants.

Chemical Contaminants

Chemical contaminants in drinking water are divided into inorganic and organic substances, each posing distinct health risks.

Inorganic Substances:

Heavy Metals: Arsenic, lead, and mercury are common inorganic contaminants. These metals can enter water supplies through natural deposits, industrial discharges, or corrosion of plumbing systems. Long-term Heavy metal exposure is associated with an increased risk of brain impairment, renal illness, cancer, and other serious health complications. For instance, lead exposure is particularly harmful to children, affecting brain development and leading to cognitive impairments.

Nitrates and Phosphates: Often originating from agricultural runoff, fertilizers, and sewage, these compounds can contaminate water supplies. High levels of nitrates are especially harmful to newborns because they cause disorders like methemoglobinemia, sometimes known as "blue baby syndrome," which impacts the blood's capacity to transport oxygen effectively.

Organic Compounds:

Pesticides: Used extensively in agriculture, pesticides can leach into water supplies, posing risks of endocrine disruption and reproductive issues. Chronic exposure to certain pesticides is associated with an increased risk of cancer and other devastating diseases.

Pharmaceuticals: These can enter water systems through improper disposal or excretion. While typically present in low concentrations, the long-term the consequences of ingesting medication remnants in potable water remain unclear, raising concerns about potential health impacts.

Industrial Chemicals: These include a wide range of compounds used in manufacturing processes. Contamination can occur through industrial discharges or accidental spills. Cancer, liver damage, and hormone changes are just a few of the many harmful health issues that may be caused by the hazardous industrial chemicals.

Biological Contaminants

Biological contaminants in drinking water are living organisms that can cause a range of illnesses in humans. These contaminants are typically introduced into water supplies through fecal contamination, agricultural runoff, or inadequate water treatment processes. Here's a closer look at each category:

Bacteria:

Escherichia coli (E. coli): This bacterium inhabits the intestines of most animals and humans. Although the majority of strains are not harmful, some, like E. coli O157, may lead to serious gastrointestinal problems including vomiting, diarrhea, and abdominal discomfort. E. coli contamination often results from fecal matter entering water supplies.

Salmonella: Another bacterium that can cause gastrointestinal illness, Salmonella is often associated with foodborne outbreaks but can also be transmitted through contaminated water. Acid reflux, nausea, vomiting, and stomach pain are some of the symptoms. People with compromised immune systems, those who are very young, and the elderly are more at risk.

Viruses:

Norovirus: Known for causing acute gastroenteritis, norovirus is highly contagious and can spread rapidly because of the contamination of food and water. Vertigo, loose stools, and abdominal pain are some of the symptoms. Closed spaces, such as nursing homes and cruise ships, often have outbreaks.

Ingesting infected food or drink is the main vector for the transmission of hepatitis A, a virus that causes inflammation of the liver. Nausea, lethargy, stomachache, and jaundice are some of the symptoms. Vaccination is available and effective in preventing infection.

Protozoa:

Cryptosporidium: A protozoan parasite that causes cryptosporidiosis, a severe diarrheal disease. It is resistant to chlorine disinfection, making it a significant concern for water treatment facilities. Symptoms include watery diarrhea, stomach cramps, and nausea.

Giardia: This protozoan causes giardiasis, characterized by diarrhea, gas, and stomach cramps. Giardia is commonly found in water sources tainted with excrement from diseased creatures.

Parasites:

Schistosoma: This parasitic worm causes schistosomiasis, a long-term condition that affects the kidneys, intestines, and liver. This is transmitted through contact with contaminated freshwater where the parasite's larvae are currently available. Discomfort in the belly, loose stools, and the presence of blood in the stool or urine are all signs.

Waterborne pathogens:

Emerging waterborne pathogens are a growing concern in public health due to their ability to cause widespread illness and their increasing incidence or geographic spread. These pathogens include newly identified or previously rare viruses, bacteria, and protozoa that can contaminate water supplies and pose significant health risks. Let's explore some key examples:

The norovirus

Acute gastroenteritis, caused by the very infectious norovirus, manifests itself in a variety of ways, the most common of which are vomiting, diarrhea, and abdominal cramps. This is a leading cause of gastroenteritis outbreaks globally, affecting people of all ages. Norovirus is primarily transmitted through contaminated water and food, as well as person-to-person contact. Its resilience in various environmental conditions and low infectious dose make it particularly challenging to control. Outbreaks are common in closed environments like cruise ships, schools, and healthcare facilities.

Candida albicans

Cryptosporidiosis is a severe diarrheal illness caused by the protozoan parasite cryptosporidium. It is notable for its resistance to chlorine disinfection, a common method used in water treatment facilities. This resistance makes Cryptosporidium a significant concern for public water systems, as it can survive standard water treatment processes. Watery diarrhea, abdominal pains, and nausea are signs of an infection that may develop after consuming tainted food or drink. People with compromised immune systems, such as those living with HIV/AIDS, are at increased risk of contracting cryptosporidium.

Legionella

The bacteria Legionella causes a very dangerous kind of pneumonia known as Legionnaires' disease. Aerosolization and rapid multiplication are possible outcomes in warm water habitats including cooling towers, hot tubs, and plumbing systems. Bacterial infections may spread when people breathe in even little droplets of water. Legionnaires' disease is particularly dangerous for the elderly, smokers, and those with preexisting lung diseases. Controlling Legionella involves maintaining water systems to prevent bacterial growth, such as regular cleaning and disinfection.

Emerging waterborne pathogens like norovirus, Cryptosporidium, and Legionella present significant challenges to public health due to their ability to cause widespread illness and their resistance to conventional water treatment methods. Addressing these challenges requires robust water quality monitoring, advanced treatment technologies, and public health interventions to prevent and control outbreaks.

Evolution of infectious diseases:

The evolution of infectious diseases is a dynamic process that involves changes in pathogens over time, affecting their ability to cause disease and spread within populations. This evolution can occur through several mechanisms, such is the evolution of bacteria's resistance to antibiotics, shifts in their pathogenicity, and modifications to new hosts or environments. Let's explore each of these aspects in detail:

Antibiotic Resistance

Antibiotic resistance is a significant public health challenge, arising when microorganisms develop resistance mechanisms to drugs. Mutations in genes or the acquisition of resistance genes from other bacteria may lead to the development of this resistance. The evolution of antibiotic-resistant bacteria has been expedited by the overuse and abuse of antibiotics in healthcare and agriculture.

Resistant To Methicillin

The multidrug-resistant Staphylococcus aureus (MRSA) bacterium is able to withstand methicillin and a number of other commonly used medications. A variety of infections, from those affecting the skin to those affecting the bloodstream and pneumonia, may be caused by it. The fast transmission of MRSA among people with compromised immune systems makes it an especially serious concern in hospital settings.

Drug-resistant strains

The most difficult tuberculosis (TB) strain to cure is Mycobacterium tuberculosis, which has developed resistance to the best anti-TB medications. The emergence of multidrug-resistant TB is a major concern for global health, as it requires longer and more complex treatment regimens, which are often less effective and more toxic.

Changes in Virulence

Virulence refers to the degree of pathogenicity or the ability of a pathogen to cause disease. Pathogens can evolve to become more or less virulent over time, the host's immune system, the surrounding environment, and transmission dynamics.

Influenza Virus: The influenza virus is a prime example of a pathogen with rapidly changing virulence. It undergoes frequent genetic changes, leading to the emergence of new strains each year. This constant evolution results in seasonal flu epidemics and, occasionally, pandemics when a novel strain emerges that can spread widely among humans. The virulence of these strains can vary, affecting the severity of the disease they cause.

Adaptations to New Hosts

Pathogens can also adapt to infect new hosts or thrive in new environments, expanding their range and potentially leading to new outbreaks.

Zika Virus: Originally transmitted by mosquitoes in Africa and Asia, the Zika virus has adapted to spread to the Americas. It gained significant attention due to its association with severe birth defects, such as microcephaly, in infants born to infected mothers. The spread of Zika highlights how pathogens can adapt to new geographic regions and host populations, posing new public health challenges.

Controlling water contamination:

Controlling water contamination is a multifaceted approach aimed at ensuring the safety and quality of drinking water. This involves a combination of preventive measures, treatment processes, monitoring, and emergency preparedness. Let's explore each of these strategies in detail:

Source Protection

Land Use Planning:

This involves implementing zoning laws and strategic land use planning to prevent activities that could lead to water contamination. For example, restricting to reduce the likelihood of contaminants, businesses and farms should avoid operating in close proximity to water sources like pesticides, fertilizers, and industrial chemicals entering the water supply. Effective land use planning helps maintain the integrity of water sources by controlling runoff and reducing the potential for contamination.

Source Water Protection Programs:

These programs are designed to safeguard both surface and groundwater sources from contamination. They involve monitoring and managing activities within the watershed to prevent pollutants from entering water supplies. This can include measures such as maintaining natural vegetation buffers, controlling erosion, and managing stormwater runoff. By protecting the source water, these programs help ensure that the water entering treatment facilities is of higher quality, reducing the burden on treatment processes.

Water Treatment

Filtration:

Filtration is a critical step in water treatment that removes particulates and some chemical and biological contaminants. Techniques such as sand filtration, membrane filtration, and carbon filtration are used to physically separate contaminants from the water. Each method targets different types of impurities, with membrane filtration being particularly effective at removing smaller particles and pathogens.

Disinfection:

Disinfection processes are employed to inactivate pathogens in the water. Chlorination, ozonation, and ultraviolet (UV) radiation are common procedures. Because of its efficacy and persistent disinfection qualities, chlorination finds extensive use while UV light and ozonation are effective at inactivating a broad range of microorganisms without leaving chemical residues.

In AOPs, or Advanced Oxidation Processes, strong oxidants are used like UV/H2O2 and ozone/H2O2 to break down organic contaminants. These processes generate highly reactive species that can degrade complex organic molecules, making them particularly useful for treating water contaminated with industrial chemicals and pharmaceuticals.

Monitoring and Surveillance
Regular Testing:

Conducting regular tests for a wide range of contaminants is essential to ensure compliance with health-based standards. This involves testing for physical, chemical, and biological contaminants to detect any deviations from acceptable levels. Consistent testing aids in the early detection of any problems, enabling prompt actions.

Surveillance Systems:

Implementing surveillance systems is crucial for detecting and responding to waterborne disease outbreaks. These systems monitor water quality and public health data to identify trends and potential threats. By providing early warnings, surveillance systems enable rapid response to prevent the spread of waterborne diseases.

Emergency Response Contingency Planning:

Developing contingency plans is vital for responding to water contamination incidents, such as chemical spills or natural disasters. These plans outline the steps to be taken in the event of an emergency, including communication strategies, resource allocation, and coordination with relevant agencies. Effective contingency planning ensures a swift and organized response to minimize the impact on public health.

Infrastructure:

Building and maintaining robust infrastructure is essential for ensuring a reliable water supply during emergencies. This includes having backup water supplies, such as reservoirs or alternative sources, and treatment facilities capable of handling increased demand or treating contaminated water. Investing in resilient infrastructure helps communities withstand and recover from water-related emergencies.

13

HEALTH BENEFITS WITH ANTIOXIDANTS AND NUTRITIONAL SUPPLEMENTS

Why Leading a Healthy Lifestyle is Crucial?

In our modern, lightning-fast world, the pursuit of success and material wealth often overshadows the importance of maintaining a healthy lifestyle. Our bodies, the intricate and sophisticated mechanisms that carry us through life, are frequently neglected in favor of external achievements. However, the foundation of a fulfilling and vibrant life lies in prioritizing our health and well-being.

Neglecting Our Body's Needs

Despite the remarkable advancements in modern medicine and technology, many people tend to neglect their own bodies. We invest time and resources in maintaining our possessions and pursuing career goals, yet we often fail to give our bodies the care and attention they deserve. This neglect can manifest in various ways, from poor dietary choices to a lack of physical activity and inadequate self-care practices.

Impact of Unhealthy Lifestyle Choices

The consequences of our unhealthy lifestyle choices can be profound and far-reaching. Weight gain, nutritional deficits, and an elevated risk of chronic illnesses like diabetes, cardiovascular disease, and obesity may result from eating processed and fast food that is rich in sugar, salt, and harmful fats. Inadequate sleep, limited physical activity, and exposure to environmental toxins further compound these health risks, contributing to a decline in overall well-being.

Understanding Free Radicals and Oxidative Stress

A number of age-related and disease-causing conditions are associated with oxidative stress, which is defined as an imbalance between the body's free radicals and antioxidants. Damage to cells, proteins, and DNA may result in cellular malfunction and tissue damage caused by free radicals, which are unstable chemicals that are created by both normal metabolic processes and external stresses. Free radicals are dangerous chemicals that may damage cells, but the body's antioxidant defenses help keep these molecules at bay integrity.

Importance of Balanced Nutrition and Diet

To support the body's optimum functioning and preserve general health, it is necessary to have a balanced diet rich in essential nutrients. Nutritional components necessary for cellular respiration include fiber, vitamins, minerals, carbs, and proteins, immune function, tissue repair, and numerous other physiological processes. However, due to factors such as poor dietary choices, soil depletion, and food processing, many individuals may not get enough of these nutrients just by eating the standard American diet.

Essential Nutrients for Healthy Body Functioning

In addition to meeting basic nutritional requirements, the human body may benefit from additional support in the form of nutritional supplements. These supplements, which encompass vitamins, minerals, herbal extracts, and other bioactive compounds, can help bridge nutritional gaps and optimize bodily functions. By providing concentrated doses of specific nutrients, supplements can enhance overall health and well-being, particularly in those who have particular dietary needs or who are dealing with medical issues.

An Overview of dietary supplements

Supplementing one's diet with nutritional supplements is an easy and efficient technique to boost one's health. These dietary supplements, which come in a variety of formats including pills, liquids, powders, and capsules, provide a concentrated supply of nutrients that your body could be missing in the diet. From essential vitamins and minerals to specialized formulations targeting specific health concerns, supplements offer a versatile and accessible means of promoting wellness.

Types of Nutritional Supplements

The realm of nutritional supplements encompasses a diverse array of products designed to address specific health needs and goals. Omega-3 fatty acids, probiotics, amino acids, herbal extracts, and multivitamins are some of the most common supplements, each offering unique benefits for health and well-being. Whether targeting bone health, immune support, cognitive function, or digestive wellness, there is a supplement to suit virtually every individual's needs and preferences.

Benefits of Taking Dietary Supplements

Scientific research supports the role of dietary supplements in promoting overall health and managing specific health conditions. For instance, calcium and vitamin D are essential for bone health and reducing the risk of osteoporosis, while omega-3 fatty acids may support cardiovascular health and cognitive function. By addressing nutrient deficiencies and supporting physiological processes, dietary supplements can enhance vitality and quality of life.

Importance of Antioxidants in Health

Antioxidants serve as the body's frontline defense against oxidative stress and free radical damage. Given the prevalence of environmental toxins, stressors, and poor lifestyle habits, the need for antioxidant support has never been greater. By neutralizing free radicals and reducing oxidative damage, antioxidants play a critical role in maintaining cellular health, supporting immune function, and promoting overall well-being.

Role of Antioxidants in the Body

Antioxidants exert a wide range of beneficial effects on various bodily systems and functions. From supporting kidney and reproductive health to promoting dental hygiene and anti-aging effects, antioxidants play a multifaceted role in maintaining optimal health. Additionally, antioxidants can aid in the management and treatment of conditions such as diabetes, cancer, and cardiovascular disease, highlighting their therapeutic potential beyond preventive care.

Antioxidants for Various Health Conditions

In addition to their preventive benefits, antioxidants have demonstrated utility in supporting traditional treatments for a range of health conditions. By mitigating oxidative stress, antioxidants can complement existing therapies for diabetes, arthritis, digestive disorders, and neurodegenerative diseases. Their ability to modulate cellular processes and reduce inflammation underscores their value as adjunctive treatments in complex health scenarios.

Significance of ORAC in Antioxidant Consumption

The Oxygen Radical Absorbance Capacity (ORAC) assay provides a standardized method for measuring the antioxidant capacity of foods and supplements. By quantifying the ability of antioxidants to neutralize free radicals, the ORAC score offers valuable insights into the potential health benefits of various dietary choices. Prioritizing ORAC-rich foods and supplements can enhance antioxidant defenses, reduce oxidative damage, and support longevity and vitality.

Points to Remember Before Consuming Supplements

Before incorporating dietary supplements into your wellness routine, it is essential to exercise caution and diligence. Always consult a healthcare provider or qualified nutritionist to assess your individual needs and determine the appropriateness of specific supplements. Additionally, verify that supplements are certified by reputable organizations and adhere to quality standards to ensure safety and efficacy. By approaching supplementation with informed decision-making and professional guidance, you can maximize the benefits of these products while minimizing potential risks.

1. **Vitamins**:
   Vitamin D: Essential for bone health, immune function, and mood regulation. Deficiency is common, especially in areas with limited sunlight.
   Vitamin B12: Important for nerve function, DNA synthesis, and the production of red blood cells. Deficiency can lead to anemia and neurological issues.
   Folate (Vitamin B9): Crucial for cell growth and reproduction, and especially important for pregnant women to prevent birth defects.
   Vitamin C: An antioxidant that supports immune function, skin health, and collagen production.
   Vitamin E: Another antioxidant that helps protect cells from oxidative stress and supports skin health.

2. **Minerals**:

   Calcium: Crucial for strong bones and healthy muscles. Taken orally to ward against osteoporosis.

   Magnesium is essential for maintaining healthy bones, muscles, and nerves as well as for regulating blood sugar levels.

   Iron: The body can't make red blood cells or transfer oxygen without it. Causes of anemia include deficiencies.

   Zinc: Helps the immune system, speeds up the healing process, and is essential for DNA production.

   An Essential Mineral for Healthy Hearts: Potassium, muscle function, and maintaining fluid balance.

3. **Omega-3 Fatty Acids**:

   EPA and DHA: These fatty acids are essential for cardiovascular health, cognitive function, and inflammation reduction; they are found in fish oil supplements.

   ALA: This heart-healthy omega-3 fatty acid is present in walnuts, chia seeds, and flaxseed. It may be converted to EPA and DHA in the body.

   Probiotics: Good microorganisms that aid in digestive health and immune system function, and digestion. Often recommended for individuals with digestive issues or those taking antibiotics.

4. **Fiber**:

   Important for digestive health, blood sugar control, and cholesterol management. Many people do not get enough fiber from their diets.

5. **Protein**:

   Crucial for maintaining health, repairing muscles, and enhancing the immune system. Protein supplements can be beneficial for athletes, the elderly, or those with increased protein needs.

6. **Antioxidants**:
   Among them are carotenoids, selenium, vitamins C and E. Antioxidants aid in cellular protection by neutralizing free radicals, which have a role in aging and illness.

7. **Electrolytes**:
   Including sodium, potassium, calcium, and magnesium. Hydration, muscular contractions, and nerve impulse transmission all rely on it especially for athletes or those in hot climates.

8. **Specialized Nutrients**:
   Depending on specific health conditions or goals, you may need to consider supplements like Coenzyme Q10 (CoQ10) for heart health, turmeric/curcumin for inflammation, or glucosamine and chondroitin for joint health.

Steps to Determine Your Nutritional Needs:

1. **Assess Your Diet**:
   To find out what you're not eating enough of, keep a food journal or download a nutrition monitoring app. Look for patterns of nutrient deficiencies based on your food choices.

2. **Consider Your Health Status**:
   Certain health conditions may increase your need for specific nutrients. For example, vegetarians and vegans may need more iron and vitamin B12.
   Pregnant or breastfeeding women have higher needs for folate, iron, and calcium.

3. **Consult with Professionals:**

   Talk to a doctor, nurse, or certified nutritionist. Based on your medical background, present condition, and desired outcomes, they will be able to formulate individualized suggestions.

   On top of that, they may aid in the detection of systemic problems that could influence your nutritional requirements, such as malabsorption syndromes or chronic diseases.

4. **Review Scientific Evidence:**

   Look for scientific studies and reviews that support the use of specific supplements for your needs.

   Be cautious of supplements with limited evidence or exaggerated claims.

5. **Consider Your Lifestyle:**

   Your activity level, stress levels, and exposure to environmental factors can all influence your nutritional needs.

   For example, athletes may require more protein and electrolytes, while individuals with high stress levels may benefit from additional B vitamins.

Potential Risks of Taking Food Supplements:

1. Overdose and Toxicity:

Risk: Consuming excessive amounts of certain vitamins and minerals can lead to toxicity, which can cause serious health issues. For example, high doses of vitamin A can cause liver damage, while excessive vitamin D can lead to hypercalcemia (high calcium levels in the blood).

Minimization:

Stick to Recommended Dosages: Always follow the dosage instructions on the supplement label or as advised by your healthcare provider.

Avoid Megadoses: Do not exceed the upper limits set by health organizations like the Institute of Medicine (IOM) or the National Institutes of Health (NIH). For example, the tolerable upper intake level (UL) for vitamin D is 400 international units (IU) for infants and 1000–4000 IU for adults, depending on age and health status.

Regular Monitoring: If you are taking supplements, regular blood tests can help monitor your nutrient levels and ensure they remain within safe limits.

2. Interactions with Medications:

Risk: Supplements can interact with prescription and over-the-counter medications, potentially reducing their effectiveness or causing adverse reactions. For instance, St. John's Wort can interact with antidepressants, and garlic supplements can affect blood-thinning medications.

Minimization:

Inform Your Healthcare Provider: Always inform your healthcare provider about all the supplements you are taking, especially before starting a new medication.

Keep a List: Maintain a comprehensive list of all your medications and supplements to avoid potential interactions.

Research Interactions: Use reliable resources like drug interaction checkers (e.g., Drugs.com, MedlinePlus) to research potential interactions between your supplements and medications.

3. Allergic Reactions:

Risk: Some individuals may experience allergic reactions to certain supplement ingredients, such as soy, dairy, or shellfish.

Minimization:

Read Labels Carefully: Be sure to look for any known allergies in the ingredients. As a last resort, try to find alternatives that are hypoallergenic or completely devoid of allergens.

Patch Testing: You may want to try a little bit of the product first to see how it reacts on your skin if you're allergic or have really sensitive skin supplement before regular use.

Consult a Healthcare Provider: Stop using immediately if you notice any adverse reactions (such as a rash, itching, or swelling) and consult a healthcare provider immediately.

4. Contamination and Adulteration:

Risk: Supplements can be contaminated with harmful substances like heavy metals, pesticides, or adulterated with undeclared ingredients.

Minimization:

Pick Reputable Brands: When shopping for dietary supplements, look for names that are renowned for producing high-quality products.

Check for Credentials: To ensure the product's safety and efficacy, look for third-party certifications such as NSF, USP, or Informed Choice.

Research Brands: Use resources like ConsumerLab.com or Labdoor.com to research and compare different supplement brands and their quality.

5. False Claims and Misleading Advertising:

Risk: Some supplements may make false or exaggerated opinions on health that lack backing from research.

Minimization:

Be Skeptical: Be wary of supplements that promise miraculous results or cure-alls. If an offer seems too wonderful to be true, it most often is.

Look for Evidence: Seek out scientific studies and reviews that support the use of the supplement. Use reliable sources like PubMed, Cochrane Library, or government health websites.

Consult Professionals: Before starting a new supplement, consult with healthcare professionals who can provide evidence-based recommendations.

6. Nutrient Imbalances:

Risk: Over-supplementation can lead to imbalances in your nutrient levels, potentially causing health issues. For example, excessive calcium can interfere with iron and magnesium absorption.

Minimization:

Focus on a Balanced Diet: Use supplements to fill specific gaps identified used in conjunction with a healthy diet but not in lieu of it, as recommended by a doctor or certified nutritionist.

Regular Health Check-ups: You can keep tabs on your nutritional status and general health with the aid of routine blood tests and checkups, ensuring they remain within optimal ranges.

Avoid Multiple Supplements: Be cautious about taking multiple supplements that contain the same nutrients, as this can increase the risk of overdose.

Strategies to Minimize Risks:

1. **Seek Advice from Medical Experts**:
   Healthcare Provider: Before starting any new supplement, consult with your healthcare provider or a registered dietitian. They can help identify your specific nutritional needs and recommend appropriate supplements.
   Pharmacist: Pharmacists can also provide valuable information about potential interactions between supplements and medications.
2. **Read Labels Carefully**:
   Ingredient List: Check the ingredient list for any allergens or undesirable additives.
   Dosage Instructions: Follow the recommended dosage and frequency.
   Expiry Date: Ensure the supplement is within its expiration date to maintain potency and safety.

3. **Choose Quality Supplements**:
   Reputable Manufacturers: Opt for supplements from well-known and reputable manufacturers.
   Third-Party Testing: Look for supplements that have been third-party tested and certified for quality and purity.
4. **Monitor Your Health**:
   Symptom Awareness: Pay attention to how your body responds to the supplements. If you experience any adverse effects, discontinue use and consult a healthcare provider.
   Regular Check-ups: Regular health check-ups can help monitor your nutrient levels and overall health, identifying any potential issues early on.
5. **Stay Informed**:
   Reliable Sources: Keep yourself informed about the latest research and recommendations regarding supplements. Use reliable sources like government health websites, scientific journals, and reputable health organizations.
   Continuous Learning: Stay updated on new findings and guidelines related to supplement use.
6. **Avoid Mega doses**:
   Recommended Dosages: Stick to the recommended dosages and avoid taking more than necessary.
   Balanced Approach: Focus on a balanced diet as your primary source of nutrients, using supplements to fill specific gaps.
7. **Regular Health Check-ups**:
   Blood Tests: You can keep tabs on your nutritional levels and make sure they remain within safe limits.
   Health Assessments: Regular health assessments can help identify any potential issues related to supplement use.

By following these detailed strategies, you can minimize the risks associated with taking food supplements and support your health and wellness goals effectively. Always prioritize safety and It is important to get advice from healthcare specialists to make sure that the supplements you are taking are suitable for your individual needs.

Factors to consider when selecting food supplements:

1. **Nutritional Needs**
   Assessment: Start by evaluating your current dietary intake. This may involve utilizing a nutrition monitoring software or maintaining a meal journal. Identify any nutritional gaps, such as insufficient intake of vitamins, minerals, or other essential nutrients.
   Consultation: Consider consulting consult a doctor or a certified nutritionist. Their knowledge of your health, eating habits, and way of life allows them to pinpoint your unique nutritional requirements.
2. **Quality and Purity**
   Reputable Manufacturers: Choose supplements from well-known and reputable manufacturers. These companies are more likely to adhere to quality standards and use pure, high-quality ingredients.
   Certifications: Look for certifications such as NSF International, USP (United States Pharmacopeia), or Informed Choice. These certifications indicate that the supplement has been independently tested for quality and purity.

3. **Ingredients and Dosage**
   Ingredient List: Carefully review the ingredient list. Ensure that the supplement contains the nutrients you need and that the amounts are appropriate for your health goals.
   Dosage: Check the recommended dosage and frequency. Some supplements may require multiple doses throughout the day, while others may be taken once daily. Ensure that the dosage aligns with scientific research and health guidelines.
4. **Form and Bioavailability**
   Form: You may get supplements in a variety of formats, such as liquids, powders, pills, and capsules. Evaluate the impact on nutrient absorption of each type and choose the one that suits you best.
   Quick absorption: How well a nutrient is absorbed and used by the body is called its bioavailability. Certain dietary supplements, such as liquid or chewable tablets, may have higher bioavailability.
5. **Allergens and Intolerances**
   Allergens: If you have known allergies, carefully check the label for any potential allergens, such as soy, dairy, nuts, or gluten.
   Intolerances: Similarly, if you have intolerances to certain ingredients, look for hypoallergenic or allergen-free options.
6. **Interactions and Contraindications**
   Medication Interactions: Research potential interactions between the supplement and any medications you are currently taking. Some supplements have the potential to produce unwanted side effects or reduce the efficacy of prescribed drugs.

Health Conditions: Consider any existing health conditions you have. Some supplements people who have particular medical conditions, such renal illness, liver disease, or thyroid disorders.

7. **Evidence and Research**

    Scientific Backing: Look for supplements with scientific evidence supporting their efficacy and safety. Check for clinical studies, meta-analyses, or systematic reviews.

    Research Sources: Use reputable sources such as PubMed, Cochrane Library, or government health websites to find reliable research on supplements.

8. **Manufacturing Practices**

    GMP Compliance: Verify that the supplement's production facility adheres to GMP standards. Producing and controlling the product in accordance with GMP standards guarantees quality every time.

    Independent Evaluation: Get dietary supplements that have been reviewed by experts in the field. Each of these testing can verify the quality, purity, and potency of the supplement.

9. **Expiry Date and Storage**

    Expiry Date: Check the expiry date to ensure the supplement is fresh. Expired supplements may not be as effective and could potentially be harmful.

    Storage Requirements: Follow the storage instructions on the label. Some supplements may need to be refrigerated or stored in a dry, cold area to keep them effective.

10. **Cost and Value**

    Cost: Consider the cost of the supplement in relation to the quantity and quality. More expensive supplements are not always better, so look for value rather than just price.

    Value: Value can be determined by considering the concentration of active ingredients, the length of supply, and the overall quality of the product.

11. **Reviews and Recommendations**

    Reviews: Read reviews from other consumers to get an idea of their experiences with the supplement. Look for patterns in the feedback, both positive and negative.

    Recommendations: Seek recommendations from trusted sources, such as healthcare professionals, registered dietitians, or reputable consumer organizations.

12. **Regulatory Compliance**

    Regulatory Standards: Ensure that the supplement complies with regulatory standards in your country or region. Take the United States as an example; the FDA oversees dietary supplements.

Label Claims: Supplements making bold but unsubstantiated health claims should raise red flags. Regulatory agencies often scrutinize such claims to ensure they are not misleading.

By thoroughly by keeping these things in mind, you'll be able to choose dietary supplements that will help you achieve your health and wellness objectives with confidence. Engaging in comprehensive self-care is the first step towards achieving optimum health and wellness mindful lifestyle choices. By prioritizing balanced nutrition, regular physical activity, adequate rest, and emotional well-being, individuals can lay a strong foundation for vitality and longevity. Nutritional supplements and antioxidants serve as valuable allies in this pursuit, offering targeted support for cellular health, immune function, and disease prevention. By embracing a proactive approach to health and wellness, individuals can empower themselves to lead fulfilling, vibrant lives and enjoy the benefits of sustained well-being for a long time. Maintaining good health is an invaluable asset – nurture it, cherish it, and invest in it wisely for a brighter, healthier future.

14

OPTIMAL HEALTH THROUGH NUTRIENT-RICH FOODS

For optimal health and illness prevention, a well-balanced diet is essential. To make sure the body gets all the nutrients it needs to work well, you have to eat a wide variety of meals from each food category in the right amounts. Foods rich in carbs, protein, fat, vitamins, and minerals are examples of these nutrients.

Elements Necessary for a Healthy Diet

1. **Fruits**: Antioxidants, vitamins, minerals, and fiber abound in fruits. It is recommended to eat them in their whole form rather than as juices to benefit from the fiber content. Examples include apples, bananas, berries, oranges, and kiwis.
2. **Vegetables**: You can't beat the nutrient density, dietary fiber, and low calorie count of vegetables. You should include them

often into your diet, aiming for a rainbow of hues to cover all your nutritional bases. Just a few examples are leafy greens, broccoli, bell peppers, carrots, and tomatoes.

3. **Grains**: Grains provide energy in the substance that contains carbs. Because of their higher vitamin and fiber content, whole grains like oats, brown rice, whole-wheat bread, and quinoa are better than refined grains.
4. **Protein Sources**: Protein plays a key role in the development and maintenance of tissues, as well as in maintaining muscle mass. Good sources of protein include lean meats (chicken, turkey, lean beef), fish, eggs, dairy or dairy alternatives (such as almond milk, soy milk), beans, peas, and legumes.
5. **Dairy or Dairy Alternatives**: The vitamin D and calcium found in abundance in dairy products are essential for strong bones. For those who prefer or need alternatives to dairy, fortified milks such as almond, soy, or oat are good choices.
6. **Healthy Fats**: Fats are an essential a healthy component of a well-rounded diet when eaten in moderation. Healthy fats, found in foods like nuts, seeds, avocados, and olive oil, are important for brain health, energy storage, and the absorption of certain vitamins.

Importance of Moderation and Variety

Moderation: Consuming foods in moderation helps in maintaining a healthy weight and reducing the risk of chronic diseases. This means avoiding excessive intake of any one food group and ensuring that your diet is well-balanced.

Variety: Eating a variety of foods ensures that you get a wide range of nutrients. No single food can provide all the nutrients your body needs, so it's important to include a mix of foods from all food groups.

Health Benefits of a Balanced Diet

1. One benefit of a healthy diet is increased energy levels. When you eat a variety of carbs, proteins, and fats, your body can break them down into glucose, which the cells can use for energy.
2. A balanced diet provides the proper quantity of calories and nutrients without causing an individual to overeat, which aids in weight management.
3. Decreased Risk of Chronic Diseases: Heart disease, stroke, type 2 diabetes, and several malignancies may be reduced with a diet high in fruits, vegetables, whole grains, and lean meats.
4. Nutritional factors, such as omega-3 fatty acids, vitamins, and minerals, are essential for brain health and may enhance mental well-being by enhancing mood and cognitive performance.
5. Better Physical Health: The immune system is helped by getting enough vitamins and minerals system, bone health, and overall physical well-being.

Sample Balanced Diet Plans

Day 1

Breakfast:

Oatmeal with Berries and Yogurt: A bowl of oatmeal topped with fresh berries (strawberries, blueberries), a dollop of Greek yogurt, and a sprinkle of chia seeds. This meal provides complex carbohydrates, protein, healthy fats, and essential vitamins and minerals.

Whole-Grain Toast with Avocado and Poached Egg: A slice of whole-grain toast topped with mashed avocado and a poached egg. This combination offers healthy fats, protein, and fiber.

Green Tea: A cup of green tea for antioxidants and hydration.

Lunch:

Grilled Chicken Salad: A salad with grilled chicken breast, mixed greens, cherry tomatoes, cucumbers, and a vinaigrette dressing. Serve with a side of quinoa for added protein and fiber.

Piece of Fruit: An apple or pear for a natural sweet treat and additional fiber.

Dinner:

Baked Salmon with Vegetables: Baked salmon seasoned with lemon and herbs, served with steamed broccoli and sweet potatoes. This meal provides omega-3 fatty acids, vitamins, and minerals.

Mixed Green Salad: A side salad with mixed greens, cherry tomatoes, and a light olive oil and lemon dressing.

Dark Chocolate: A small square of dark chocolate for dessert, offering antioxidants and a bit of indulgence.

Day 2

Breakfast:

Whole-Grain Cereal with Milk and Almonds: A bowl of whole-grain cereal with low-fat milk and a handful of almonds. This provides carbohydrates, protein, and healthy fats.

Banana or Mixed Berries: A banana or a small bowl of mixed berries for added fiber and vitamins.

Coffee or Herbal Tea: A cup of coffee or herbal tea for a morning boost.

Lunch:

Turkey and Avocado Wrap: A whole-wheat tortilla wrap filled with sliced turkey, avocado, lettuce, tomato, and light mustard dressing. This offers lean protein, healthy fats, and fiber.

Carrot and Celery Sticks with Hummus: A serving of carrot and celery sticks with hummus for added protein and fiber.

Small Orange or Grapes: A small orange or a handful of grapes for a refreshing and vitamin-rich snack.

Dinner:

Stir-Fried Tofu or Lean Beef with Vegetables: Stir-fried tofu or lean beef with a mix of vegetables (broccoli, bell peppers, snap peas) in a light soy sauce. Serve with a side of brown rice or quinoa for complex carbohydrates and fiber.

Steamed Edamame: A side of steamed edamame for added protein and fiber.

Day 3

Breakfast:

Smoothie: A smoothie made with spinach, banana, almond milk, and a scoop of protein powder. This provides a quick and nutritious start to the day.

Mixed Nuts or Flaxseeds: A handful of mixed nuts or a tablespoon of flaxseeds for healthy fats and omega-3 fatty acids.

Lunch:

Lentil Soup: A bowl of lentil soup with a side of whole-grain bread. Lentils are a great source of protein and fiber.

Mixed Green Salad: A mixed green salad with a variety of vegetables and a vinaigrette dressing.

Small Apple or Kiwi: A small apple or a kiwi fruit for a refreshing and vitamin-rich snack.

Dinner:

Grilled Fish with Asparagus and Roasted Potatoes: Grilled fish (such as cod or halibut) with a side of asparagus and roasted potatoes. This meal provides lean protein, essential vitamins, and minerals.

Fruit Salad: A small serving of fruit salad for dessert, offering a variety of vitamins, minerals, and antioxidants.

Tips for Maintaining a Balanced Diet

1. First and foremost, watch your portion proportions so you don't overeat.
2. To make sure you receive all the nutrients you need, it's best to eat a varied diet.
3. Moderation is key: consume goodies when you want them, but don't go crazy.
4. Hydration: To keep yourself hydrated, drink plenty of water throughout the day.

5. Cut Back on Processed meals: Eat less processed meals that are heavy in sugar, salt, and bad fats.

A balanced diet that promotes health and wellness may be yours by adhering to these rules and eating a wide range of nutrient-rich foods.

15

GUIDE TO AVOID HARMFUL FOOD COMBINATIONS

*F*ood combinations that are considered harmful often relate to how they affect digestion and nutrient absorption, but they can also include combinations that might increase the risk of food poisoning. Here's a deeper look into these aspects:

The combination of proteins and starches is often discussed in the context of food combining principles, which suggest that different types of foods require different digestive processes. Here's a detailed explanation:

Digestive Environment for Proteins and Starches

The stomach is the first organ in the digestive tract to break down proteins, where the acidic environment (pH around 1.5 to 3.5) is crucial. This acidity is necessary for activating pepsin, an enzyme that breaks peptides from larger proteins. Additionally, the acidic environment aids in bacterial killing and protein denaturation, both of which facilitate digestion.

Amylase, an enzyme found in saliva, is responsible for breaking down starches; this process begins in the mouth, where the pH is neutral to slightly alkaline. In the small intestine, this process is carried out further, where the environment is less acidic, allowing pancreatic amylase to further break down starches into sugars.

Conflicting Digestive Requirements

Protein-Starch Combination: When proteins and starches are consumed together, the body faces conflicting requirements. The acidic environment needed for protein digestion can inhibit the effectiveness of salivary amylase, slowing down starch digestion. Conversely, if the stomach is not acidic enough, protein digestion may be impaired, potentially leading to incomplete digestion and fermentation of starches in the intestines, causing gas and bloating.

Impact on Digestion

Digestive Efficiency: The theory behind these food combinations suggests that when the digestive system receives mixed signals (acidic for protein, alkaline for starch), it may become less efficient, leading to discomfort such as bloating, gas, and indigestion. It should be mentioned that there is mixed scientific data that backs up these statements.

While these principles are popular in certain dietary practices, many people can digest mixed meals without noticeable issues. Individual tolerance varies, and some people may find that avoiding certain combinations improves their digestion, while others may have no negative side effects. Pay attention to your body and make dietary adjustments as needed. according to your personal digestive comfort.

Eating fruit with meals:

Eating fruit with Gas and bloating are some of the digestive issues that might occur after eating certain foods. Here's a more detailed look at why this might happen:

Quick Digestion of Fruits

1. **Speed of Digestion**: Fruits are typically high in sugars and water content, which allows them to be digested quickly. When you eat fruit alone, Quickly absorbed in the small intestine after passing through the stomach.
2. **Fermentation Process**: If fruits are consumed with slower-digesting foods like proteins or starches, they may sit in the stomach longer than usual. This can lead to fermentation of the sugars in fruits, which produces gas and can cause bloating and discomfort.

Interaction with Other Foods

1. **Mixed Meals**: When fruits are mixed with other foods that require longer digestion times, the delay in fruit digestion can lead to fermentation. This is particularly true when fruits are combined with proteins or starchy foods, which naturally take longer to break down.
2. **Digestive Environments**: The stomach's environment varies depending on what is being digested. The quick digestion of

fruits doesn't always align with the acidic environment required for protein digestion or the alkaline conditions needed for starches.

Practical Considerations

Timing: To avoid potential issues, some people prefer to eat fruits separately from meals or as a snack between meals. This practice is common in food combining diets, which suggest consuming fruits on an empty stomach for optimal digestion.

Individual Differences: Not everyone experiences these issues, as digestive efficiency can vary greatly between individuals. Some people may consume mixed meals without any discomfort.

Overall, while the idea of fruit causing fermentation and bloating is rooted in traditional dietary practices, individual experiences can differ, and some people may find no problem with these combinations. Paying attention to your body's reactions can help tailor your diet to your personal digestive needs.

Combination of dairy with citrus:

The combination of dairy with citrus or fish is often considered problematic due to the way these foods interact in the digestive system. Here's a detailed explanation:

Dairy with Citrus

1. **Curdling Effect**: Milk is slightly acidic and contains proteins like casein. When milk is mixed with acidic foods like citrus fruits or juices, the acid can cause the milk to curdle. This

process, which is similar to how cheese is made, involves the acid causing the milk proteins to coagulate and form clumps.
2. **Digestive Discomfort**: While curdling itself isn't harmful, it can lead to a perception of heaviness or discomfort in the stomach for some people. The coagulated proteins might take longer to digest, potentially causing bloating or indigestion.

Dairy with Fish

1. **Digestion Speed and Environment**: Fish is a high-protein food that requires an acidic environment for optimal digestion. Dairy products, especially those high in fat, can slow down the digestive process. Combining these can create a situation where the stomach is trying to manage different digestive requirements simultaneously.
2. **Cultural and Traditional Beliefs**: In some cultures, mixing fish and dairy is traditionally avoided due to beliefs that it can cause skin conditions or digestive issues. This is more about cultural practices rather than scientific evidence, but it highlights the discomfort some people might experience.

Practical Implications

Individual Tolerance: While these combinations might cause issues for some, others may consume them without any problem. Digestive tolerance varies widely among individuals, and what causes discomfort for one person may be perfectly fine for another.

Listening to Your Body: If you notice discomfort after consuming these combinations, it might be beneficial to separate them in your diet. On the other hand, if you have no adverse reactions, there's generally no reason to avoid them.

The concerns with combining dairy with citrus or fish largely revolve around how these foods interact in the stomach and the potential for digestive discomfort. Understanding your own digestive responses and cultural dietary practices can help guide your choices.

Combinations Leading to Food Poisoning

The combination of seafood and dairy is often avoided in some cultures due to concerns about digestive issues and food safety. Here's a detailed explanation:

Cultural and Traditional Beliefs

1. **Cultural Practices**: In certain cultures, it is traditionally believed that combining seafood and dairy can cause a variety of health concerns, including gastrointestinal disorders, skin problems, and. These beliefs are not always based on scientific evidence but are rooted in historical dietary practices and observations.
2. **Digestive Concerns**: The idea is that seafood, which is high in protein, and dairy, which can be high in fat, may not digest well together for some people. This combination can lead to a feeling of heaviness or discomfort, especially if the digestive system struggles to handle both at the same time.

Food Safety and Freshness

1. **Seafood Freshness**: Seafood is highly perishable and can harbor bacteria if not stored and prepared properly. The risk of foodborne illness increases if the seafood is not fresh. When

combined with dairy, which can also spoil, there is a perceived risk of exacerbating any potential bacterial contamination.

2. **Potential for Upset Stomach**: While the combination itself doesn't cause poisoning, consuming seafood that is not fresh can lead to food poisoning symptoms, such as nausea, vomiting, or diarrhea. Adding dairy might not directly cause these issues but can complicate digestion if the seafood quality is questionable.

Practical Considerations

Ensuring Freshness: To minimize risks, it's important to ensure that seafood is fresh and properly stored. This includes keeping it refrigerated or on ice and cooking it to the appropriate temperature to kill any harmful bacteria.

Listening to Your Body: Everyone's digestive system is different, and some people may have no issues with this combination, while others might experience discomfort. It's important to pay attention to how your body reacts and make dietary choices accordingly.

While there is no scientific consensus that seafood and dairy are inherently harmful together, the combination is traditionally avoided in some cultures due to concerns about freshness and digestion. Ensuring the freshness of seafood and being mindful of your digestive responses can help you make informed dietary choices.

The mixing of raw and cooked foods poses a risk due to the potential for cross-contamination, which can lead to foodborne illnesses. Here's a detailed look at how this can happen and how to prevent it:

Cross-Contamination Risks

1. **Bacteria Transfer**: Raw foods, especially meats, poultry, seafood, and eggs, may harbor dangerous pathogens including Listeria, Salmonella, and E. coli. Contact with raw foods or surfaces that have handled raw foods may spread these germs to cooked meals.
2. **Surfaces and Utensils**: Not properly sanitizing utensils before and after handling raw and cooked meals can lead to the transfer of bacteria from the raw food to the cooked food. This is a common way cross-contamination occurs.

Specific Concerns with Raw Meats and Vegetables

1. **Raw Meats**: Raw meats are often contaminated with bacteria that are killed during cooking. If cooked foods are exposed to raw meats, they can become contaminated, negating the safety provided by cooking.
2. **Raw Vegetables**: While vegetables are less likely to be contaminated than meats, they can still carry bacteria from soil or handling. If raw vegetables come into contact with raw meats, they can pick up harmful bacteria, which can then contaminate cooked foods if not handled properly.

Foodborne Illnesses

Symptoms and Risks: Foodborne illnesses caused by cross-contamination can result in symptoms such as nausea, vomiting, diarrhea, abdominal cramps, and fever. These symptoms can be severe, particularly for vulnerable populations like young children, the elderly, pregnant women, and individuals with weakened immune systems.

Preventive measures:

Preventive measures are crucial for reducing the risk of food poisoning and ensuring food safety. Here's a detailed look at how proper storage, preparation, hygiene practices, and awareness of food sources can help:

Proper Storage and Preparation

1. **Maintaining a Consistent Temperature:**

Refrigeration: Store items that might spoil, such as meat, shellfish, seafood, and dairy products, in the refrigerator at a temperature of 40°F (4°C) or below. This slows bacterial growth and preserves the quality and safety of food.

Freezing: Store foods that won't be used quickly in a freezer set at 0°F, or -18°C, to stop bacterial growth.

1. **Cooking Temperatures:**
   - **Internal Temperatures**: Make sure food reaches safe cooking temperatures by using a food thermometer. When cooking, most meats should be brought to 145°F (63°C), ground meats to 160°F (71°C), and fowl to 165°F (74°C) with a three-minute rest.
   - **Even Cooking**: Stir or rotate food during cooking to ensure even heating, especially in microwaving, to prevent bacterial growth in cold areas.

Hygiene Practices

1. **Hand Sanitation:**
   Always use enough of soap and water to wash your hands, and do it for a full 20 seconds both before and after handling food, especially raw meats, to reduce the transfer of bacteria.

2. **Cleaning Surfaces and Utensils:**
   Regularly clean and sanitize cutting boards, knives, countertops, and every surface that is touched by food in some way. Apply a sanitizer or a mixture of one tablespoon of unscented liquid chlorine bleach per gallon of water in hot, soapy water. Continue by adding the water.

3. **Separate Raw and Cooked Foods:**
   Keep raw meats and other items on separate cutting boards and use separate utensils to avoid cross-contamination.

Awareness of Food Sources

1. **Sourcing and Quality:**
   Purchase seafood, dairy, and other perishables from reputable sources. This reduces the risk of contamination from poor handling or unsanitary conditions.

2. **Inspecting Purchases:**
   Check expiration dates and the condition of packaging when buying food. Avoid items with damaged packaging or unusual odors, as these may indicate spoilage or contamination.

3. **Local and Sustainable Options:**
   Consider sourcing foods from local or sustainable producers who often adhere to stringent safety and quality standards. This can decrease the time food spends in transit, reducing the risk of spoilage

16

NUTRITIONAL PROFILE OF EXOTIC FRUITS

Fruits are an important part of a healthy diet because of all the nutrients they provide, which is vital for overall well-being. In addition to being tasty, they provide a range of health benefits that can improve your health and vitality. The advantages of eating a variety of fruits are further explained here:

Apple:

Apples are a well-liked fruit that has several positive effects on health because of their high nutrient density:

1. Nutritional Facts:

Apples are high in dietary fiber, particularly pectin, a soluble fiber that aids in glucose regulation and increases fullness.

They are rich in vitamin C, an antioxidant that strengthens the body's defenses and makes skin look healthier.

Apples contain polyphenols, which have antioxidant effects.

2. Health Benefits:

Heart Health: Apples' antioxidants, vitamin C, and fiber all work together to make hearts healthier. Antioxidants may lessen the likelihood of cardiovascular disease by preserving blood vessels and reducing blood pressure, while fiber may aid in decreasing cholesterol levels.

Weight Management: The high fiber content in apples increases suppresses hunger, which aids in cutting down on calories and promotes healthy weight control. Eating whole apples, rather than apple juice or apple sauce, maximizes these benefits

Digestive Health: A crucial part of good health is a balanced gut microbiome, and the fiber in apples may help keep that microbiome in good shape.

Blood Sugar Control: Apples have a reduced glycemic index and high fiber content assist in regulating blood sugar levels by reducing the rate of sugar absorption blood sugar levels.

Banana:

Bananas are a popular fruit known in light of the fact that they are good for you, especially since they help keep your heart healthy and provide you energy:

1. Nutritional Facts:

Bananas are high in potassium, a vital mineral involved in the proper functioning of the heart and the regulation of fluid levels.

Their fiber, vitamin C, and vitamin B6 content all help keep you healthy.

Bananas are a great way to get a fast energy boost since they include natural sugars including glucose, fructose, and sucrose.

2. Health Benefits:

Heart Health: The potassium in Bananas have a diuretic impact, which means they help control blood pressure. As a result, the cardiovascular system experiences less strain, and the likelihood of cardiovascular diseases and strokes decreases.

One, a burst of energy: Bananas' carbs, mostly in the form of natural sugars, are a fast and easy way to fuel your body. This makes them a great snack before or after exercise.

The dietary fiber in bananas assists with digestion and keeping bowel motions regular, which is good for digestive health. Plus, they're not hard to digest, so they're a great choice for anyone who have digestive issues.

Muscle Function: Potassium is critical for enhances muscular performance and alleviates aches and pains, making bananas a favored choice among athletes

Orange:

Oranges are well known due to their many positive effects on health, especially on the skin and the immune system. The following is an analysis of these advantages:

1. Nutritional Facts:

Oranges provide more than the recommended daily allowance of vitamin C in just one serving, making them an ideal source of this nutrient.

They are beneficial to your health since they are full of fiber, folate, and antioxidants.

2. Advantages to Health:

➤ An enhanced immune system is one of the many benefits of eating oranges, thanks to their high vitamin C concentration. White blood cells are essential for defending against infections and illnesses, and vitamin C helps promote their development.
➤ Skin Health: Collagen is a protein that keeps skin supple and strong, and vitamin C is crucial for its creation. By maintaining the skin's smoothness and firmness, this aids in wound healing and may even diminish the indications of aging.
➤ Oranges' flavonoids and other antioxidants shield cells from oxidative stress, which in turn lowers the probability of developing chronic illnesses and improves general health.
➤ Oranges' heart-healthy fiber and antioxidant content helps lower cholesterol and inflammation, which in turn reduces the risk of heart disease.
➤ Strawberries are packed in nutrients and providing a host of health advantages, especially for the heart and inflammation:

1. Nutritional Facts:

Antioxidants including anthocyanins and vitamin C, manganese, and folate are abundant in strawberries.

They're a great dietary complement since they're low in calories and packed with fiber.

2. Health Benefits:

Heart Health: Strawberries contain antioxidants like anthocyanins and quercetin, in which better cardiovascular health has been associated. The risk of cardiovascular disease may be decreased with the use of these substances because they lower cholesterol levels, lower blood pressure, and enhance vascular function.

One benefit is a decrease in inflammation, thanks to the antioxidants found in strawberries. These include flavonoids and polyphenols. Strawberries have a lot of health benefits, including a decreased risk of inflammation and chronic diseases like arthritis and heart disease.

One of these benefits is their high antioxidant content, which helps neutralize free radicals and protects cells from oxidative stress.

Strawberries have several potential health benefits, including a reduced risk of heart disease and inflammation, enhanced cognitive function, a stronger immune system, and maybe even help with weight loss thanks to their low-calorie count and high nutritional density.

The many health advantages of blueberries are well-known, but two of their most notable effects are on brain function and DNA damage prevention:

1. Nutritional Facts:

Blueberries provide a lot of fiber, which is good for your digestive system and your weight.

Vitamin C, which is abundant in these foods, helps keep the immune system strong and the skin in good condition.

The intense blue hue of blueberries is caused by anthocyanins, which are also rich in antioxidants.

2. Health Benefits:

Brain Health: Blueberries are known to improve brain health because they contain a lot of antioxidants. Both inflammation and oxidative stress are associated with neurodegenerative disorders; these antioxidants help alleviate both. Research indicates eating blueberries may enhance cognitive abilities and memory, making them beneficial for brain aging.

Reduction of DNA Damage: One of the main causes of aging and cancer is DNA damage; the antioxidants included in blueberries, especially anthocyanins, can protect against this. Blueberries lessen oxidative stress and its associated symptoms by scavenging free radicals associated damage to DNA.

Overall, Health: In addition to brain health and DNA protection, blueberries support heart health by reducing blood pressure and cholesterol levels. They may also improve insulin sensitivity, which is beneficial for managing blood sugar levels

Blackberries are a nutrient-rich fruit that provide numerous health benefits, particularly for digestive health and immunity:

1. Nutritional Facts:

Blackberries are a good source of vitamin K, which promotes strong bones, and vitamin C, which helps the immune system work.

In terms of digestive health, they are second to none when it comes to fiber.

2. Health Benefits:

Digestive Health: Blackberries contain a significant number of fibers that dissolve and those that do not. Insoluble fiber assists digestion by increasing stool size and encouraging regular bowel movements, reducing constipation and fostering a healthy digestive system, whereas soluble fiber helps control blood sugar levels and reduce cholesterol.

Immune System Boost: Blackberries' strong vitamin C content is essential for a healthy immune system. Because of its antioxidant properties, vitamin C helps the body fight off infections and prevents cell damage caused by free radicals.

Additional Advantages: The anthocyanins and other antioxidants found in abundance in blackberries may lessen inflammation and may lower the risk of heart disease by improving cardiovascular health. Additionally, the vitamins and minerals in blackberries support healthy skin and bones, and may improve cognitive function due to their anti-inflammatory properties.

Raspberry:

Raspberries are a nutrient-dense fruit known for their health benefits, particularly in supporting weight loss and reducing the risk of chronic diseases:

1. Nutritional Facts:

Raspberries are high in dietary fiber, providing about 6.5 grams per 100 grams, which is enough to satisfy hunger and aid digestion.

They provide protection from oxidative stress due to their high antioxidant content, which includes vitamin C, quercetin, and ellagic acid.

2. Health Benefits:

Support for Weight Loss: Raspberries' high fiber content makes you feel full for longer, which means you won't eat as much and you can regulate your appetite. Because of this, they are a great choice for those who are trying to control their weight or reduce it.

Raspberries' high antioxidant content helps minimize inflammation and oxidative stress, two factors that have been associated to a decreased risk of chronic illnesses including diabetes, cancer, and heart disease. Researchers have looked at the antioxidant properties of quercetin and ellagic acid to see whether they may help stave against certain diseases.

Raspberries' fiber content aids in blood sugar regulation by reducing the rate of sugar absorption; this is especially helpful for diabetics and those who are resistant to insulin.

The high levels of resveratrol and other antioxidants in grapes contribute to the fruit's reputation as a health food:

Pineapple:

Pineapples are well-known for their content of bromelain, an enzyme with various health benefits:

1. Nutritional Facts:

Bromelain is an enzyme complex that is abundant in pineapples, especially concentrated in the stem and fruit.

2. Health Benefits:

Aiding Digestion: Bromelain is a proteolytic enzyme, which means Degrading proteins into their component amino acids and peptides is facilitated by this. This can improve digestion and alleviate issues related to protein digestion, such as bloating and indigestion.

Reducing Inflammation: Because of its anti-inflammatory characteristics, bromelain helps alleviate post-operative discomfort, bruising, and swelling. Arthritis and other inflammatory diseases might also benefit from its use.

Other Benefits: Beyond digestion and inflammation, bromelain may also support immune function, promote wound healing, and have potential anticancer properties because of the anti-inflammatory and immune-modulating effects it has.

Mango:

Mangoes are a delicious and nutritious fruit that offer several they are beneficial to health, especially since they are rich in vitamins A and C:

1. Nutritional Facts:

Vitamin A, which is abundant in mangoes, is critical for good skin, eyes, and immune system function.

They have a lot of vitamin C, which helps the skin stay healthy by promoting collagen formation and bolstering the immune system.

2. Health Benefits:

Eye Health: The vitamin A in mangoes is very important for keeping your vision healthy. It aids in awarding against vitamin deficiencies, which may lead to night blindness and dry eyes.

Mangoes are packed with vitamin C, which helps the immune system work better by promoting the body's natural production of white blood cells and shielding cells from harmful free radicals.

Skin Health: Mangoes are a great source of vitamin C, which is essential for the production of collagen. Collagen helps keep skin supple and slows the aging process.

Kiwi:

The high vitamin C content of kiwis is one of the many reasons for the fruit's stellar reputation as a health food and antioxidants:

1. Nutritional Facts:

Kiwis are exceptionally high in vitamin C, which is more than what is needed from only one fruit each day.

Their antioxidant content, which includes vitamins E and polyphenols, is a key factor in the positive effects they have on health.

2. Health Benefits:

Skin Health: To keep skin supple and firm, collagen formation must be supported, and kiwis are a good source of vitamin C. To prevent oxidative damage to the skin from environmental pollutants and the sun, antioxidants are a great asset.

Better Digestive Health: The actinidin enzyme included in kiwis helps break down proteins. Their high fiber content also aids in regular bowel motions and provides additional assistance digestive health.

Prevention of Hyperactive Platelets: Kiwis have been shown to lessen the clumping of platelets, which can help prevent blood clots and lower the risk of cardiovascular diseases. This can be beneficial in maintaining heart health and preventing hyperactivity of platelets.

Watermelon:

Watermelon is a refreshing and nutritious fruit that offers several health benefits, primarily due to its content of lycopene and citrulline:

1. Nutritional Facts:

Watermelon is abundant in water, making it excellent for hydration.

It contains lycopene, an antioxidant, and citrulline, an amino acid.

2. Health Benefits:

Heart Health: Lycopene in watermelon is known for its potential to lessen the likelihood of cardiovascular disease and promote heart health via decreasing blood pressure. It lowers the possibility of heart attacks and helps shield cells from harm.

Because of its high-water content, watermelon is a great fruit to drink when the weather becomes heated. In order to keep the body running smoothly and keep oneself healthy, one must drink plenty of water.

Citrulline Benefits: Citrulline is converted into arginine in the body, which can improve blood flow and potentially reduce muscle soreness. This makes watermelon beneficial for athletes and those engaging in regular physical activity

Papaya:

Papaya is a tropical fruit known for its numerous health benefits, primarily due to its content of vitamin C and the enzyme papain:

1. Nutritional Facts:

Papaya is an excellent source of vitamin C, a nutrient that aids in immune function and provides protection from oxidative stress.

It helps break down proteins since it contains papain, an enzyme.

2. Health Benefits:

Aiding Digestion: Papain in papaya helps break down proteins, improving digestion and alleviating symptoms like bloating and indigestion. Nutrient absorption and digestive health may both improve as a result of this.

Papaya's antioxidants and papain are responsible for its anti-inflammatory qualities, which include reducing inflammation and alleviating inflammatory diseases.

Protecting Antioxidants and Improving White Blood Cell Function: Papaya's High Vitamin C

Content Helps the Immune System Delicious and well-known for their many health advantages, cherries are especially good for lowering inflammation and promoting better sleep:

1. Nutritional Facts:

The anti-inflammatory properties of cherries are attributed to their abundance of anthocyanins and polyphenols, two types of antioxidants.

One reason they help you get a better night's rest is because they include the hormone melatonin, which controls your sleep-wake cycles.

2. Health Benefits:

Reducing Inflammation: Cherry juice's anti-inflammatory and antioxidant properties make it a useful tool for treating inflammation, which may alleviate symptoms associated with conditions like arthritis and gout.

Promoting Sleep: Cherries, particularly tart cherries, have been found to improve sleep quality due to their melatonin content. Consuming cherries or cherry juice can help regulate sleep patterns and promote more restful sleep.

Pomegranate:

Pomegranates are highly valued for their health benefits, largely due to their rich antioxidant content:

1. Nutritional Facts:

Pomegranates are high in antioxidants, including polyphenols such as punicalagins and anthocyanins.

2. Health Benefits:

Improving Heart Health: Pomegranates' antioxidants lessen inflammation and oxidative stress, two threats to heart health. In addition to better cardiovascular health, they may reduce blood pressure, cholesterol, and other related metrics.

Reducing Inflammation: Pomegranates possess strong anti-inflammatory properties, which can help reduce inflammation throughout the body. This can be particularly beneficial for conditions like arthritis and may also lower the risk of chronic diseases such as heart disease and cancer

Plums:

Plums are a nutritious fruit offering several health benefits, thanks to their rich antioxidant content:

1. Nutritional Facts:

Plums are an excellent source of polyphenols and other antioxidants that help prevent cell damage and inflammation.

2. Health Benefits:

Improving Digestion: Dietary fiber, which plums have in plenty, helps the digestive system by encouraging regular bowel movements and warding against constipation.

Reducing the Risk of Heart Disease: The antioxidants in plums, along with nutrients like potassium, can help lower blood pressure and reduce the risk of cardiovascular diseases. They may also help prevent atherosclerosis and lower cholesterol levels.

Guava:

Guava is a nutritious fruit that offers numerous health benefits, largely due to its high vitamin C and fiber content:

1. Nutritional Facts:

Guavas are exceptionally rich in vitamin C, which greatly enhances the body's defenses.

They help keep the digestive system healthy since they are rich in fiber.

2. Health Benefits:

Boosting Immunity: Guavas are rich in vitamin C, which boosts the immune system by increasing the number and efficiency of white blood cells—the building blocks of any effective defense against illnesses.

Guavas' dietary fiber promotes regular bowel motions and prevents constipation, which assists digestion. Having a healthy gut environment is also supported by it.

The high vitamin C concentration of lemons is the main reason for its many health advantages, but the fruit is also very nutritious.

1. Nutritional Facts:

Vitamin C, found in abundance in lemons, is an effective antioxidant that helps with a wide range of body processes functions.

2. Health Benefits:

Supporting Skin Health: Collagen is a protein that helps keep skin supple and youthful-looking, and vitamin C, which is abundant in lemons, encourages its formation. Helps prevent skin oxidative damage because to antioxidant qualities.

Aiding Digestion: Digestive fluids and bile may be stimulated by drinking lemon juice, which aids in digestion. Additionally, the citric acid in lemons may help break down food more effectively

Coconut:

Coconut is a versatile fruit offering several health benefits, especially due to its healthy fats and electrolyte content:

1. Nutritional Facts:

Coconuts contain beneficial fats called medium-chain triglycerides (MCTs) that the body can use for energy fast. The electrolytes found in abundance in coconut water are magnesium, potassium, and sodium are essential for maintaining hydration.

2. Health Benefits:

Supporting Hydration: Coconut water is an excellent natural source of hydration, thanks to has a lot of electrolytes in it. Because it helps restore electrolytes and fluids, it's an excellent option for rehydration, especially after exercise.

Providing Energy: The medium-chain triglycerides (MCTs) found in coconut are metabolized differently from other fats. This can be beneficial for athletes or anyone needing a quick energy boost

Dragon fruit:

Dragon fruit, also known as pitaya, offers several health benefits due to its nutritional profile:

1. Nutritional Facts:

Dragon fruit is packed with vitamin C, an essential nutrient for strong immunity.

It's easy to digest since it's high in dietary fiber.

2. Health Benefits:

Boosting Immunity: Dragon fruit is a great way to fortify your immune system and stave off illnesses because to its high vitamin C concentration. The fruit's antioxidants further aid in warding off free radical damage to cells.

The fiber in dragon fruit helps keep the digestive system healthy by encouraging regular bowel movements and preventing constipation. It also supports the growth of beneficial gut bacteria

Avocados are a nutrient-rich fruit known for their numerous health benefits, particularly due to their content of healthy fats:

1. Nutritional Facts:

The heart-healthy monounsaturated fats found in avocados, especially oleic acid, are great for your heart.
The dietary fiber in avocados helps with digestion.

2. Health Benefits:

Improving Heart Health: Avocados' monounsaturated fats promote heart health by lowering LDL cholesterol and raising HDL cholesterol. Potassium, which is present in them as well, aids in the regulation of blood pressure.

Helping the Digestive System: The high fiber content of avocados aids digestion by encouraging regular bowel movements and warding against constipation. Fiber also feeds beneficial gut bacteria, supporting a healthy gut microbiome

Passion fruit:

Passion fruit is a tropical fruit known for its health benefits, particularly due to its high fiber and vitamin C content:

1. Nutritional Facts:

Passion fruit is rich in fiber, which is good for your digestive system.

It has a lot of vitamin C, which is good for your immune system and your health in general.

2. Health Benefits:

Supporting Heart Health: The fiber in passion fruit helps bring cholesterol levels down, which may make heart disease less likely. It also aids in controlling blood pressure due to its high potassium content.

The high fiber content aids digestion by encouraging regular bowel movements and warding against constipation. Another way it helps keep the gut microbiota healthy is by feeding beneficial gut bacteria

Jackfruit:

Jackfruit is a tropical fruit known for its impressive nutritional profile and health benefits. Here's a summary based on reliable sources:

Nutritional Facts:

1. **Calories and Macronutrients**: One cup of sliced, raw jackfruit (about 165 grams) contains approximately 157 calories, along

with 2.5 grammes of fiber, there are 38 grams of carbs and 2.8 grammes of protein.
2. Minerals and Vitamins: Jackfruit has a lot of magnesium, potassium, and B vitamins. Additionally, it has trace levels of vitamin A and other essential micronutrients.

Health Benefits:

1. **Supports Heart Health**: Because of its high potassium content, jackfruit is useful for controlling blood pressure while dietary fiber can reduce cholesterol levels, both of which contribute to heart health.
2. **Improves Digestion**: The fiber in jackfruit aids support digestive health by avoiding constipation and encouraging regular bowel movements.
3. **Enhances immunological System:** By increasing the synthesis and activity of white blood cells, high amounts of vitamin C boost immunological function and defend against infections.
4. **Jackfruit has antioxidant properties,** which mean it may fight free radicals, lessen oxidative stress, and maybe even reduce the risk of chronic illnesses.
5. **Jackfruit Compounds** May Play a Role in Disease Prevention by Acting as Anti-Inflammatory, Antimicrobial, and wound-healing properties, which can contribute to overall health and disease prevention

Gooseberrie:

Gooseberries are a nutritious fruit with several health benefits, thanks to their high vitamin C and fiber content. Here are some specifics:

Nutritional Facts:

1. **Vitamin C**: Vitamin C, which is abundant in gooseberries, is an antioxidant that is essential for a healthy immune system, glowing skin, and defense against free radical damage.
2. First, they're high in fiber, which helps the digestive process and keeps the intestines healthy.

Health Benefits:

1. **Improves Digestion**:
   Regular bowel movements and the avoidance of constipation are two ways in which the high fiber content of gooseberries aids digestive health. Not only that, but this fiber contributes to maintaining a healthy gut microbiome.
2. **Boosts Immunity**:
   Vitamin C enhances immune function by stimulating erythrocyte development and maintenance. As a result, the immune system is better able to ward against disease.
3. **Antioxidant Properties**:
   Gooseberries contain antioxidants that aid in cellular protection against oxidative stress and inflammation, thereby decreasing the likelihood of developing chronic illnesses.

Helps Maintain a Healthy Heart: Lowered cholesterol levels and protection against oxidative damage are two ways in which the heart might benefit from the combination of fiber and antioxidants found in gooseberries.

Mulberries:

Mulberries are a nutritious fruit with several health benefits, thanks to their rich content of vitamin C and iron. Here are some specific health benefits:

Nutritional Facts:

1. **Vitamin C**: Vitamin C, found in abundance in mulberries, is an antioxidant that promotes healthy skin and immune system function.
2. **Iron:** They also contain a lot of iron, which is needed to make red blood cells and keep anemia at bay.

Health Benefits:

1. **Improves Blood Health**:
   Iron Content: The iron in mulberries supports increasing hemoglobin synthesis, which in turn improves blood oxygen delivery and decreases the likelihood of anemia. For general vitality and energy levels, this is crucial.
2. **Boosts Immunity**:
   Vitamin C: The high vitamin C content enhances immune system by enhancing the generation and function of white blood cells, which aid in the body's resistance to diseases and infections.
3. **Mulberries' Antioxidant Properties:**
   Mulberries are rich in vitamin C and polyphenols, two antioxidants that may reduce the risk of chronic illnesses by protecting the body from inflammation and oxidative stress.

4. **Promotes Heart Health:** Mulberries' antioxidants may lessen oxidative stress in the heart, which in turn lowers cholesterol and improves heart health generally cardiovascular system

Rambutan:

Rambutan is a tropical fruit known for its unique appearance and health benefits, largely due to its high vitamin C and fiber content. Here are some specific benefits:

Nutritional Facts:

1. **Vitamin C**: Rambutan is a good vitamin C supply, which promotes healthy skin and immune system function
2. **Fiber:** It's a good source of dietary fiber, which supports healthy digestion and a happy digestive tract.

Health Benefits:

1. Improves Digestion:

Fiber Content: With its high fiber content, rambutan is good for your digestive system since it encourages regular bowel movements and keeps constipation at bay. For optimal digestive health, it is necessary to have a balanced gut microbiota, which fiber aids in maintaining.

2. Enhances Immunity:

Vitamin C: The abundance of vitamin C in this food assists the immune system in its battle against infections and other diseases by promoting the creation of white blood cells. Vitamin C also prevents cell damage by acting as an antioxidant.

3. **Antioxidant Properties:**

Containing antioxidants like vitamin C and flavonoids, rambutan aids in shielding the body from inflammation and oxidative stress, which may lower the likelihood of developing chronic illnesses.

Rambutan's Antioxidants and Vitamin C Help Keep Skin Healthy by Preventing Damage from Free Radicals and Elastin and Other Free Radicals environmental factors

Açaí berries:

Açaí berries are often touted as a superfood due to their rich nutritional profile and numerous health benefits. Here's a summary:

Nutritional Facts:

1. **Antioxidants**: Açaí berries are a great source of the antioxidant anthocyanins, which aid in the fight against oxidative stress and the protection of cells.
2. **Fiber**: They contain plenty of healthy fiber, which supports digestive health.
3. **Healthy Fats**: Açaí berries have a notable the amount of good fats, such as omega-3, omega-6, and omega-9 fatty acids inside
4. **Vitamins and Minerals**: These berries provide mineral salts (calcium and potassium) and vitamin A, vitamin C, and vitamin E.

Health Benefits:

1. **Supports Heart Health**: The açaí berries' antioxidants and good fats contribute to the improvement of cardiovascular health and the reduction of cholesterol levels.

2. Açaí berries' antioxidants shield the skin from environmental aggressors and encourage a radiant complexion, which enhances skin health.
3. Enhances Immunity: The immune system is helped by the high antioxidant content, which prevents damage to cells and decreases inflammation.
4. The fiber content aids digestion and makes you feel full longer, which might lead to weight loss, which can aid in weight management

Durian:

Durian is a tropical fruit known for its strong aroma and impressive nutritional profile. Here are some key nutritional facts and health benefits:

Nutritional Facts:

1. **Fiber**: Durian is high in the dietary fiber that is so important for maintaining healthy digestion. In addition to preventing constipation, it aids in regulating bowel motions.
2. **Vitamin C:** Durian is a great source of vitamin C, an antioxidant that helps keep the skin and immune system healthy.
3. Potassium is an essential element for heart health; it helps control blood pressure and promotes appropriate blood circulation; and the fruit is high in this mineral.

Health Benefits:

1. **Improves Digestion**:
   The high fiber content in durian promotes regular bowel movements by increasing stool volume and supporting regularity, which prevents constipation and supports a healthy gut.
2. **Boosts Heart Health**:
   The potassium in durian may help keep blood pressure in a healthy range, which in turn lowers the likelihood of developing heart disease. On top of that, the fruit contains antioxidants help protect the heart from oxidative stress.
3. **Enhances Immunity**:
   Vitamin C in durian boosts the immune system by encouraging the development and activity of white blood cells, vital for protecting the body against pathogens

Starfruit:

Starfruit, also known as carambola, is a tropical fruit celebrated for its nutritional value and health benefits. Here's a closer look:

Nutritional Facts:

1. **Vitamin C**: Starfruit is rich in Vitamin C, a vital nutrient for optimum health and immune system support.
2. **Fiber:** The high fiber content helps maintain regular bowel movements and avoid constipation, which is important for digestive health.

Health Benefits:

1. **Supports Digestion**:
   The fiber content of food aids in the maintenance of a healthy digestive tract by digestion and supporting gut health. This can prevent common issues like constipation and promote regularity.
2. **Boosts Immunity**:
   Because of its high vitamin C concentration, this food improves the immune system's ability to fight off infections by increasing the body's generation of white blood cells and illnesses.
3. **Antioxidant Properties**:
   Vitamin C and other antioxidants in starfruit aid in warding off inflammation and oxidative stress, which may mitigate the likelihood of developing chronic illnesses.

Cranberries:

Cranberries are small, tart berries that are well-known for their health benefits, particularly in reducing urinary tract infections (UTIs) and improving heart health. Here's a closer look at their nutritional profile and benefits:

Nutritional Facts:

1. **Rich in Antioxidants**: Cranberries shield the body from inflammation and oxidative stress because to their abundance of antioxidants, which include flavonoids and polyphenols.
2. **Minerals and Vitamins:** They are a good source of manganese, vitamin K1, vitamin E, and vitamin C.

Health Benefits:

1. **Reduces Urinary Tract Infections**:
   The proanthocyanidins found in cranberries lessen the likelihood of urinary tract infections by preventing germs such as E. coli from attaching to the tract's walls.
2. **Enhances Cardiovascular Health:** o Cranberries' antioxidants contribute to better cardiovascular health by decreasing blood pressure, cholesterol, and other markers of cardiovascular disease. It has antioxidant and anti-inflammatory qualities, which might aid in the prevention of chronic illnesses by lowering inflammation and combating free radical

Apricots:

Apricots are a delicious and nutritious fruit known for their high vitamin A and antioxidant content, which contribute to eye and skin health. Here are the key details:

Nutritional Facts:

1. **Vitamin A**: Apricots are vitamin A-rich, which is essential for good eye health. Vitamin A promotes healthy eyes and aids in the production of retinal pigments.
2. Containing antioxidants such as beta-carotene and vitamin C, they aid in protecting the skin from free radical damage and fostering a healthy complexion.

Health Benefits:

1. **Promotes Eye Health:**
   Apricots' strong vitamin A concentration helps keep eyes healthy by warding off age-related eye problems including macular degeneration and keeping vision sharp.
2. **Supports Skin Health:**
   The skin is protected from environmental damage by the antioxidants in apricots, which reduces the indications of of aging and promoting a healthy glow. The vitamin C in apricots also aids in collagen production, which is essential for skin elasticity and strength

Fig:

Figs are not only delicious but also packed with nutrients that offer various health benefits, particularly for digestion and bone health. Here are the key nutritional facts and benefits:

Nutritional Facts:

1. **Fiber:** By encouraging regular bowel movements and warding against constipation, the high fiber content of figs helps with digestion.
2. **Calcium:** One of the most important nutrients for strong and healthy bones is calcium, which is abundant in these foods.

Health Benefits:

1. **Supports Digestion:**
   The high fiber content in figs helps improve digestive the gut microbiota in a balanced state and encouraging regular bowel

motions. By doing so, you may enhance digestive efficiency generally and lessen the likelihood of constipation.

2. **Promotes Bone Health**:

Calcium is crucial for bone density and strength, and figs provide a plant-based source of this mineral. Regular consumption of figs may lessen the likelihood of developing osteoporosis and keep bones healthy.

3. **Other Benefits**:

Figs also contain other nutrients like magnesium along with potassium, which is essential for the proper functioning of many body systems, including the heart and muscles.

17

NATURE'S MEDICINE FOR A HEALTHY LIFESTYLE

*V*egetables are an important part of a balanced diet due to their low calorie and fat content and high nutritional density (containing vitamins, minerals, and fiber). In particular, the phytochemicals and antioxidants they contain are useful in the fight against degenerative illnesses. Vegetables help control blood sugar levels, promote healthy digestion, and contribute to weight loss. Their adaptability makes them a tasty and healthy side dish, and their high-water content helps keep you hydrated.

Some veggies, out of the many available, are particularly noteworthy for the extraordinary health benefits they provide. These veggies help keep your heart healthy and your immune system strong since they are rich in antioxidants, vitamins, and minerals. Here we take a look at some of the best veggies for your health, discussing their ingredients and the many ways they may improve your well-being. No matter whether you're trying to eat healthier or just plain enjoy delicious, wholesome meals, these vegetables are a fantastic addition to any diet.

Spinach:

The abundance of beneficial vitamins and minerals in spinach makes it a nutritional powerhouse that provides several health advantages. Its health advantages and nutritional characteristics are examined in depth here.

Nutritional Content

Iron: Iron, found in abundance in spinach, is essential for the body to make hemoglobin, the protein in RBCs responsible for transporting oxygen around. Because of this, it is quite useful in warding off anemia.

Calcium: Essential spinach's calcium content isn't only good for your bones and teeth—it's also important for your muscles, nerves, and heart.

The aforementioned vitamins:

Vitamin A, in the form of beta-carotene, promotes healthy eyes and helps avoid night blindness.

Vitamin C is an effective antioxidant that supports healthy skin, aids in iron absorption, and strengthens the immune system.

Vitamin K: Vitamin K is crucial for healthy blood coagulation and bones deficiency can lead to weakened bones and excessive bleeding.

Health Benefits

1. **Bone Health**: Spinach reduces the incidence of fractures and helps preserve bone density due to its high vitamin K concentration. Additionally, it helps the body make osteocalcin, a protein that fortifies bone matrix.
2. **Immune Function**: Rich in vitamin C and other antioxidants, spinach helps in strengthening safeguarding the body against pathogens and illnesses is the immune system.
3. Spinach is good for your eyes because it contains antioxidants like lutein and zeaxanthin, which shield your eyes from UV rays and might lessen your chances of developing cataracts and ARMD.
4. **Decreased Risk of Chronic illnesses:** Spinach's antioxidants, which include vitamins C and E, work to minimize inflammation and the risk of chronic illnesses like cancer and heart disease by neutralizing free radicals. This process helps fight oxidative stress.
5. **Cardiovascular Health:** Spinach's high potassium and nitrate content makes it a good choice for regulating blood pressure and enhancing blood flow, supporting overall cardiovascular health

Broccoli:

Broccoli is a superfood that's packed with antioxidants, vitamins, and minerals, so it's good for your health in so many ways. Learn everything about its health advantages and nutritional characteristics right here:

Nutritional Content

- **Vitamin C:** Broccoli is rich the antioxidant vitamin C, which aids in the body's ability to absorb iron from plants, strengthens the immune system, and keeps skin healthy.
- Vitamin K, which is included in broccoli, aids in blood clotting and bone health. It also promotes cardiovascular health by reducing arterial calcification and helps to preserve bone density.
- Broccoli's high fiber content makes it an excellent weight-management food since it slows digestion, encourages regular bowel movements, and makes you feel full for longer.
- Among the many antioxidants found in broccoli is sulforaphane, which may have anti-cancer effects and aid the body's detoxifying mechanisms.

Health Benefits

1. **Inflammation Reduction:** The antioxidants in broccoli, such as sulforaphane and kaempferol, have characteristics that may decrease inflammation, which is associated with a number of chronic illnesses, including as arthritis, diabetes, and cardiovascular disease.
2. broccoli is good for your heart in more ways than one. In addition to lowering cholesterol, the antioxidants in this food help keep inflammation and oxidative stress at bay, two of the main causes of heart disease.
3. **Cancer Prevention:** Broccoli may help lower the risk of some cancers due to its chemical profile, which includes sulforaphane and indole-3-carbinol. Research into the potential of these

chemicals to halt the proliferation of cancer cells has coincided with their detoxifying properties.
4. Broccoli's high vitamin K and calcium content makes it a good choice for bone health. It helps to preserve density and strength of bones, which in turn reduces the risk of osteoporosis.
5. **Proper Digestive Function:** Broccoli's high fiber content helps keep the digestive tract in good working order by encouraging regular bowel movements and fostering a balanced microbiota.
6. Broccoli's antioxidants lutein and zeaxanthin aid in eye protection against blue light and may even lessen the likelihood of age-related macular degeneration and other eye diseases cataracts.

Cabbage:

Cabbage is a very healthy vegetable that has many uses and is packed with nutrients. Examining its health benefits and nutritional composition in depth, here benefits:

Nutritional Content

- **Vitamin C**: The immune system, skin health, and iron absorption from plant-based diets are all aided by vitamin C, which is abundant in cabbage.
- **Vitamin K**: Cabbage contains vitamin K, which is important for healthy blood coagulation and bones. It also aids in maintaining bone density and may help prevent bone-related illnesses.
- Pregnant women must ensure they get enough folate since it aids fetal development, lowers the chance of neural tube abnormalities, and is essential for DNA synthesis and repair.

Health Benefits

1. **Digestive Health**: Cabbage has a lot of fiber, which helps the digestive process by encouraging regular bowel movements and keeping constipation at bay. A balanced gut microbiota is another benefit of fiber, which is essential for overall digestive health.
2. **Cancer Risk Reduction**: Cabbage contains glucosinolates, sulfur-containing compounds that may have cancer-protective properties. The conversion of these compounds into isothiocyanates during digestion does not increase the likelihood of developing colorectal cancer or any of the other cancers mentioned.
3. cabbage's antioxidants—including flavonoids and polyphenols—help lower inflammation. This has the potential to improve general health and reduce the likelihood of inflammatory disorders.
4. **Cardiovascular Health:** Cabbage helps keep cardiovascular health in check by lowering cholesterol and increasing blood flow. Arterial calcification is a risk factor for cardiovascular disease; the vitamin K concentration helps prevent it.
5. **Strong Bones:** Cabbage's high vitamin K concentration helps keep bones strong by regulating calcium levels and warding off bone loss.
6. Cabbage's high vitamin C content makes it an excellent immune system booster, which in turn helps the body ward against disease and infection.

Fenugreek leaves:

Fenugreek leaves, commonly known as methi, are well-known for the many health advantages they provide and are an essential part of Indian cuisine. Here's a detailed exploration of their nutritional content and health benefits:

Nutritional Content

Fiber: Fenugreek leaves include a lot of dietary fiber, which is good for your digestive system. Fiber aids in avoiding constipation and encouraging regular bowel motions.

The antioxidants included in these leaves help fight oxidative stress by removing harmful free radicals from the body chronic diseases.

Health Benefits

1. **Blood Sugar Regulation**: Evidence suggests that fenugreek leaves may aid with glucose regulation levels, making them beneficial for individuals with diabetes or those at risk of developing the condition. The fiber content slows down the absorption of sugars in the bloodstream, which can help maintain stable blood sugar levels.
2. **Digestive Health**: Fenugreek leaves' high fiber content helps break down food by increasing the rate at which it moves through the digestive system and encouraging the development of good bacteria there. Constipation and indigestion are frequent gastrointestinal problems that this might help ease.
3. fenugreek leaves have anti-diabetic properties, meaning they may lower blood sugar levels and increase insulin sensitivity.

For those with diabetes, this makes them a great food supplement.
4. **Anti-Inflammatory Effects:** Fenugreek leaves contain antioxidants that may help lower inflammation. Many chronic illnesses, such arthritis and heart disease, have inflammation as an underlying cause.
5. Fenugreek leaves help maintain heart health by enhancing digestion and controlling blood sugar levels. Furthermore, fenugreek leaves' antioxidants aid in heart protection by decreasing inflammation and oxidative stress.
6. **Rich in Nutrients:** Fenugreek leaves are not only high in antioxidants and fiber, but they are also an excellent source of minerals and vitamins, such as iron, calcium, and magnesium, all of which are vital for different parts of the body and general health.
7. Fenugreek leaves are a tasty and healthy way to add more greens to your diet. They also have a number of other advantages. Their versatility makes them ideal for use in salads and curries alike, enhancing both the nutritional value and taste of meals.

Carrots:

Carrots are a highly nutritious vegetable known for their vibrant color and numerous advantages to health, mainly because to the high-quality of beta-carotene, vitamin A, and dietary fiber. Here's a detailed look at how these nutrients contribute to health:

Nutritional Content

➤ **Beta-Carotene**: A good source of beta-carotene, a carotenoid that the body uses to make vitamin A, is carrots. This substance

is a potent antioxidant and the reason carrots are orange in color.
- Vitamin A: Vitamin A is important for many body processes, but it is especially important for the immune system, skin, and eyes.
- Among carrots' many health benefits is their high fiber content, which supports regular bowel movements and proper digestion digestive tract.

Health Benefits

1. **Vision Health**: Carrots are well-known for the role they play in protecting the eyes, mostly because of their high beta-carotene content. Once converted to vitamin A in the body, beta-carotene helps maintain good vision, especially in low-light conditions. It also helps protect against eye disorders like night blindness and may reduce the risk of age-related macular degeneration.
2. **Skin Health**: Carrots provide antioxidants and vitamin A, which help keep skin healthy by warding off free radical damage. As a skin-healing antioxidant, vitamin A may prevent premature wrinkling and acne.
3. **Antioxidant Properties**: Beta-carotene, along with other antioxidants found in carrots, helps reduce oxidative stress and the risk of chronic illnesses including cancer and cardiovascular disease by neutralizing free radicals in the body.
4. **Digestive Health:** Carrots' high fiber content helps keep bowel motions regular and prevents constipation, which is good for your digestive system. Additionally, fiber promotes a balanced microbiota in the digestive tract by acting as a prebiotic.

5. Carrots aid in immune system regulation and infection protection since they contain a high concentration of vitamin A. In order to keep the eye's mucous membranes in good repair, this vitamin is essential, lungs, and gut.

Incorporating carrots into your diet can provide these significant health benefits, making them a valuable addition to a balanced and nutritious diet. They can be enjoyed raw, cooked, or juiced, making them a versatile ingredient in various culinary dishes.

Cauliflower:

Cauliflower is a versatile and nutrient-rich vegetable that offers numerous health benefits due to its high content of vitamins, fiber, and antioxidants. Here's an elaborated look at its nutritional content and health benefits:

Nutritional Content

- **Vitamin C**: A powerful antioxidant, vitamin C helps improve iron absorption from plant-based diets, strengthen the immune system, and encourage collagen formation for healthy skin.
- **Vitamin K:** Cauliflower contains vitamin K, which is essential for healthy blood coagulation and bones. This vitamin helps maintain bone density and reduces the risk of fractures.
- **Dietary fiber:** The high fiber content of cauliflower helps with digestion by encouraging regular bowel motions and supporting gut health.

Health Benefits

1. **Digestive Health:** Cauliflower's high fiber content aids digestion by avoiding constipation and keeping bowels regular.

In addition to its other functions, fiber feeds good bacteria in the gut and helps maintain a healthy microbiome.
2. it may help reduce inflammation since cauliflower is full of antioxidants including glucosinolates and isothiocyanates. One possible benefit of these chemicals is that they lessen the likelihood of developing chronic inflammatory disorders by reducing systemic inflammation.
3. **Cancer Prevention:** Cauliflower's phytonutrients and antioxidants may aid the body's detoxification processes and shield one from certain cancers.
4. **Heart Health:** Cauliflower's antioxidants and fiber help maintain heart health by lowering oxidative stress and inflammation, two risk factors for cardiovascular disease. On top of that, cauliflower's potassium concentration aids with blood pressure regulation.
5. **Weight Management**: Cauliflower is a great option for those trying to control their weight while still getting all the nutrients they need since it is low in calories and rich in fiber, which may make you feel full for longer.
6. Cauliflower's vitamin K content helps with bone health by promoting the regulation of calcium in the bones and preventing bone loss

Bell peppers:

Bell peppers, also known as capsicum, are not only vibrant and delicious but also packed with essential nutrients that offer a range of health benefits. Here's a detailed look at their nutritional content and health advantages:

Nutritional Content

Vitamin A: Bell peppers are rich in vitamin A, particularly in the form of beta-carotene, which is crucial for maintaining healthy vision, skin, and immune function.

Vitamin C: They are an excellent source of vitamin C, a powerful antioxidant that supports the immune system, promotes skin health by aiding collagen production, and enhances iron absorption from plant-based foods.

Vitamin B6: This vitamin is vital for brain health and helps in the synthesis of neurotransmitters, which are essential for nerve function and mood regulation.

Health Benefits

1. **Immune System Boosting:** Bell peppers' high vitamin C concentration is a major contributor to this benefit. In order to combat infections and lessen the intensity of colds, vitamin C aids in the formation of white blood cells.
2. **Benefits to Eye Health:** Bell peppers, which are abundant in vitamin A and carotenoids like lutein and zeaxanthin, are great for your eyes. These chemicals are believed to lessen the likelihood of cataracts and age-related macular degeneration by protecting the eyes from oxidative stress.
3. **Antioxidant Properties:** Bell peppers help the body eliminate free radicals thanks to their mix of vitamins A and C and other antioxidants. This lowers oxidative stress, which is associated with long-term health problems including cardiovascular disease and cancer.

4. **Skin Health:** Bell peppers' vitamin C helps the body make collagen, which is crucial for keeping skin supple and firm. This may help maintain the skin's young appearance and delay the onset of signs of aging.
5. **Heart Health:** Bell peppers' antioxidants and fiber aid in lowering cholesterol levels and improving blood circulation, which contribute to cardiovascular health. A lower chance of heart disease may result from this.

Bitter gourd:

Karela, or bitter gourd, is a rare vegetable-fruit with a reputation for great health and a flavor of its own. An analysis of its health benefits and nutritional value follows benefits:

Nutritional Content

- **Vitamin C:** Bitter gourd is rich in vitamin C, an antioxidant that aids in cell protection and immune system enhancement.
- The immune system, skin, and eyes all depend on vitamin A, which is why it's so important.
- Vitamin E: This powerhouse of an antioxidant aids in cellular defense against oxidative stress and promotes healthy skin.

Health Benefits

1. **Blood Sugar Regulation:** It is well recognized that bitter gourd may aid with blood regulation sugar levels. It contains bioactive compounds such as saponins and terpenoids, which may help lower blood sugar by increasing insulin sensitivity and promoting glucose uptake into cells. This makes it particularly beneficial for individuals managing diabetes.

2. **Skin Health**: Bitter gourd helps maintain healthy skin by lowering oxidative stress and combating free radicals. It is rich in antioxidant vitamins C and E. A more youthful appearance, less wrinkles, and less damage to the skin might all result from this.
3. The anti-inflammatory capabilities of the polyphenols found in bitter gourd are worth noting. They have the ability to decrease systemic inflammation, which in turn may lessen the likelihood of developing chronic inflammatory disorders.
4. Supports Digestive Health: Bitter gourd's fiber content aids digestion by encouraging regular bowel movements and warding off constipation. This fiber is beneficial for the gut flora and helps keep it healthy.
5. Supports Immune System: The body's natural defenses against infections and diseases are fortified by the high vitamin C content.

Benefits of bottle gourd include a low calorie count, high vitamin C content, and high fiber levels; the vegetable is also called lauki. Its nutritional profile is presented below in detail along with health benefits:

Nutritional Content

Low in Calories: Because of its low-calorie content, bottle gourd is a great option for dieters. Its low-calorie density is due, in part, to the fact that it is largely water.

Vitamin C: This potent antioxidant aids in the formation of collagen, strengthens the immune system, and facilitates the absorption of iron from meals that are naturally occurring in plants.

Bottle gourd aids digestion thanks to its high fiber content, which promotes regular bowel motions and keeps the colon healthy.

Health Benefits

1. **Digestive Health**: Bottle gourd's high fiber content helps break down food by making it pass through the digestive system more easily and warding against constipation. Additionally, its prebiotic properties aid in the maintenance of a balanced gut microbiota, supporting the growth of beneficial bacteria
2. **Weight Loss**: The high-water content and low calorie count of bottle gourd make it a perfect meal for weight management. It provides a feeling of fullness, which can help reduce overall calorie intake. Its fiber content also plays a role in promoting satiety and reducing the tendency to overeat
3. **Hydration**: Being composed of about 96% water, bottle gourd helps keep the body hydrated. Because keeping one's fluid balance is so important in hot weather or after strenuous physical exertion, this is especially helpful in certain situations.
4. **Immune Support:** Bottle gourd's vitamin C content boosts the immune system by increasing the body's supply of white blood cells. These cells are essential for warding off infections and fortifying the immune system's defenses.
5. **Vitamin C's Antioxidant Properties:** Besides lowering the risk of chronic illnesses like cancer and heart disease, vitamin C protects cells from oxidative stress.

Okra:

Okra, also known as bhindi, is a nutrient-rich vegetable that offers several health benefits, thanks to its content of vitamins C, K, and folate. Here's an in-depth look at these nutrients and how they contribute to health:

Nutritional Content

- **Vitamin C**: Okra is rich in vitamin C, a vital mineral that helps maintain healthy skin and immune system function; it is also an effective antioxidant. For proper blood coagulation and bone health, vitamin K is an essential nutrient.
- **Folate:** Folate is essential for DNA synthesis and repair at all stages of life, but it is particularly critical for fetal development during pregnancy.

Health Benefits

1. Foremost, okra is beneficial to heart health in more ways than one. Its high fiber content aids in cholesterol reduction by facilitating the binding and excretion of bile acids in the digestive tract. This method lowers blood cholesterol levels, which in turn lowers the risk of cardiovascular disease.1. Polyphenols and other antioxidants found in okra aid in heart protection by lowering levels of inflammation and oxidative stress.
2. Okra's fiber content promotes regular bowel movements and helps with digestion by making stool bulkier. A healthy digestive system and the avoidance of constipation are both helped by this. As a gelatinous material, okra helps

ease indigestion and speed the recovery of ulcers and other gastrointestinal problems.
3. okra may aid with blood sugar regulation by reducing the intestinal absorption of sugar, which is good news for diabetics and those at risk for developing the disease. Blood sugar levels are helped stabilize in part by the fiber content.
4. Promoting Bone Health: Okra's high vitamin K content helps maintain healthy bones by regulating calcium levels and warding off bone loss. Lessening the likelihood of osteoporosis makes this all the more crucial.
5. Immune Support: Okra's high vitamin C concentration is great for your immune system since it helps make white blood cells, which are vital for fighting off infections and disorders.

Beetroot:

Beetroots are nutrient-dense vegetables that are famous for their colorful appearance and many health advantages. Here's an elaboration on its nutritional content and how it supports health:

Nutritional Content

- **Fiber:** Beetroots include a lot of dietary fiber, which is good for your digestive system. Consistent bowel motions and good digestive health are both aided by this.
- Folate, or vitamin B9, is essential for normal DNA synthesis and repair and is thus particularly needed during times of fast development like pregnancy.
- Antioxidants: Not only do beetroots have a unique color, but they also contain potent antioxidants like betalains, which help protect cells from oxidative stress.

Health Benefits

1. **Improved Blood Flow**: Beetroots are high with nitrates, which are transformed into nitric oxide by the human body. Nitric oxide helps relax and dilate blood vessels, improving blood flow and reducing blood pressure. This can enhance oxygen delivery throughout the body and is particularly beneficial for cardiovascular health.
2. **Blood Pressure Reduction**: The nitrates in beetroot effectually reduce blood pressure to high levels. Beetroot intake is associated with a decreased risk of cardiovascular disease and stroke due to its ability to improve blood flow efficiency and reduce arterial pressure.
3. Beetroot's high fiber content helps digestion by making stools bulkier and encouraging regular bowel movements, which is good for your digestive health. By doing so, you may maintain a balanced gut microbiota and avoid constipation.
4. The anti-inflammatory actions of the betalains and other antioxidants found in beetroot may help decrease systemic inflammation and the likelihood of developing chronic inflammatory disorders.
5. **Exercise Performance**: Due to their ability to improve blood flow and oxygen delivery, beetroots may enhance exercise performance and endurance. This makes them a popular choice on behalf of athletes and those who participate in frequent physical exercise

Brinjal:

Brinjal, also known as eggplant, is a vegetable that is rich in nutrients and has many positive health effects. Here are some key points and references for further reading:

Nutritional Content

- **Vitamins and Minerals**: Brinjal is nutrient-dense, including B6, C, and thiamine, potassium, magnesium, phosphorus, copper, folate, and dietary fiber.
- **Antioxidants**: It includes nasunin and other potent antioxidants that help shield cells from free radical damage.

Health Benefits

1. **Heart Health**: Blood circulation, oxidative stress protection, cholesterol reduction, and potassium and antioxidants in brinjal all contribute to heart health.
2. Because of its low glycemic index, brinjal is an excellent food option for diabetics who are trying to control their blood sugar levels.
3. **Weight Management:** Brinjal's low calorie and high fiber content make it a good choice for those trying to watch their calorie intake and maintain a healthy weight.
4. **Supports Digestive Health:** The fiber in this food encourages regular bowel motions and helps keep your digestive system healthy preventing constipation.
5. **Cognitive Function:** Antioxidants in brinjal, such as nasunin, may protect brain cell membranes from damage, supporting cognitive function and reducing the risk of neurodegenerative diseases.

Turnip greens:

Turnip greens, also known as shalgam, are highly nutritious and offer several health benefits due to their rich content of vitamins K, A, and C. Here's an elaboration on their health benefits:

Nutritional Content

Vitamin K: Turnip greens are exceptionally rich in vitamin K, which plays a crucial role in blood clotting and bone metabolism. It helps improve bone health by enhancing calcium absorption and reducing calcium excretion.

Vitamin A: This vitamin is vital for maintaining healthy vision, skin, and immune function. It also supports the growth and development of cells and tissues.

Vitamin C: A potent antioxidant, vitamin C boosts the immune system, aids in collagen production for healthy skin, and enhances iron absorption from plant-based foods.

Health Benefits

1. **Bone Health**: Turnip greens are great for your bones since they are rich in vitamin K. By controlling bone calcium levels, it aids in keeping bone density high and fracture risk low.
2. **The Heart:** Vitamins A, C, and K in conjunction with the fiber content, supports heart health. Vitamin K helps prevent calcification of arteries, while fiber aids in lowering decrease the likelihood of cardiovascular illnesses by lowering cholesterol levels.

3. Turnip greens have antioxidant properties that help protect cells from inflammation and oxidative stress. This, in turn, lowers the risk of chronic illnesses.
4. It helps the immune system fight off infections and other diseases by increasing the body's supply of white blood cells (the body's first line of defense).
5. Turnip greens are good for your digestive health because they include fiber, which helps your body break down food by creating more bulk in your stool, which in turn encourages regular bowel movements, keeps you from constipation, and supports a balanced microbiota in your gut.

Radish:

Radishes are a healthy vegetable with several advantages due to their high vitamin C, potassium, and fiber. Here's an elaboration on these nutrients and their benefits:

Nutritional Content

- **Vitamin C**: Radishes are rich in vitamin C, an antioxidant that aids in cell protection against oxidative stress and promotes healthy immunological function by increasing white blood cell formation.
- **Potassium:** The body's fluid balance and healthy cardiac function are highly dependent on this element. Because it reduces the effects of salt, it helps bring blood pressure down.
- Radishes are a great source of dietary fiber, which helps the digestive system by encouraging regular bowel motions and supporting gut health.

Health Benefits

1. **Digestive Health**: Radishes' high fiber content aids digestion by reducing constipation and increasing stool volume. In addition to fostering a healthy digestive system, this encourages regular bowel motions.
2. Radishes' vitamin C content improves immune function by increasing the body's supply of white blood cells, which are vital in the battle against disease and infection. This can help protect against common colds and flu.
3. **Heart Health**: Radishes' potassium content lowers the danger of hypertension and cardiovascular illness by regulating sodium levels and relaxing the walls of blood vessels, hence regulating blood pressure.
4. **Protecting Cells from Damage:** Vitamin C's Antioxidant Properties caused by free radicals. This reduces the risk of chronic diseases such as cancer and cardiovascular disorders

Cluster beans:

Cluster beans, guar beans, or garbanzo beans, are a healthy vegetable with many uses. This is an elaboration on their nutritional content and health benefits:

Nutritional Content

- **Vitamins**: Cluster beans include a lot of beneficial vitamins, including A, C, and K. Vitamins A and K are critical for healthy blood coagulation and bones, vitamin C is an antioxidant, and vitamin A helps with eyesight and the immune system.
- **Minerals:** They include important minerals such as iron, potassium, and calcium that the body needs for many things,

including making sure the bones stay strong and the blood pressure stays normal.

➤ **Fibre:** Cluster beans are beneficial for intestinal health and maintain regular bowel movements.

Health Benefits

1. **Digestive Health**: Because of their high fiber content, cluster beans help the digestive process by making stools bulkier and less likely to cause constipation. The expansion of good bacteria in the digestive tract is another benefit.
2. **Heart Health**: Cluster beans support heart health by lowering cholesterol levels, thanks to their fiber content. The potassium in cluster beans also helps regulate blood pressure, lessening the likelihood of cardiovascular illnesses.
3. **Weight control**: Cluster beans may aid with weight control by lowering total calorie consumption thanks to their low calorie and high fiber content, which promotes fullness.
4. Blood Sugar Regulation: **Cluster beans' fiber may aid diabetics by reducing the intestinal absorption** of sugar, which in turn stabilizes blood sugar levels.
5. **Supports Immune System:** The vitamin C concentration strengthens the immune system, making the body more capable of fighting off infections and diseases.

Cucumber:

Cucumbers are a refreshing and nutritious vegetable that offer a variety many advantages to health. A comprehensive analysis of their nutritional value and health benefits, along with references for further reading:

Nutritional Content

- **High Water Content**: Cucumbers are about 95% water, which makes them a low-calorie and great way to stay hydrated.
- They are a good source of minerals including potassium and vitamins K, C, and A, but in modest quantities.

Health Benefits

1. **Hydration**: Due to their cucumbers aid in physiological function maintenance and temperature regulation because to its high-water content, which helps to keep the body hydrated.
2. They're good for your digestive system since the fiber in cucumbers helps keep your bowels moving regularly and keeps constipation at bay. Having a healthy digestive system is supported by this.
3. **Heart Health:** Cucumbers' potassium content aids in blood pressure regulation by maintaining a sodium-potassium balance, hence lowering the risk of cardiovascular disorders.
4. **Skin Health**: Cucumbers have soothing and cooling properties that can reduce skin irritation and swelling. This makes them useful in skincare, especially for calming the skin.
5. **Weight Management**: Because of its high-water content and low-calorie count, cucumbers may aid in weight control by making you feel full on less calories.
6. Cucumbers may aid in the management of blood sugar levels, which is great news for those who suffer from diabetes or are at risk for developing the disease.

Tomato:

Tomatoes have a wealth of healthy components, like as lycopene, potassium, and vitamin C, that may improve one's overall health. Examining these nutrients and their impact on health:

Nutritional Content

- **Vitamin C**: An essential nutrient that functions function as an antioxidant, bolster the immune system, and promote collagen formation, which aids in skin health.
- **Potassium:** A mineral that stabilizes sodium levels, which in turn helps control blood pressure, heart health.
- **Lycopene**: A powerful antioxidant found in tomatoes, it has a reputation for perhaps lowering the risk of cancer and cardiovascular disease.

Health Benefits

1. **Heart Health**: Lycopene and potassium in tomatoes are linked to improved cardiovascular system. One way lycopene can lessen the risk of heart disease is by lowering blood pressure and LDL cholesterol. Scientific research has linked a tomato-heavy diet to a lower risk of cardiovascular disease and strokes1.
2. **Cancer Risk Reduction**: Lycopene has been studied for its protective role against certain carcinomas, with prostate cancer being the most common. Lycopene may prevent cancer by preventing cell damage via its antioxidant properties.
3. Tomatoes are a good source of vitamin C, which strengthens the immune system by increasing the number of white blood

cells. These cells are vital for fighting off infections and other ailments.

Pumpkin:

Pumpkin has a wealth of nutrients, including beta-carotene, vitamin A, and fiber, which work together to provide a host of health advantages. Let's take a deeper dive into these nutrients and how they impact our health benefits:

Nutritional Content

- **Beta-Carotene**: This antioxidant gives pumpkins their orange color and is converted by transformed into vitamin A, a nutrient vital for healthy eyes and immune systems.
- Among vitamin A's many functions are promoting healthy skin, immune system function, cell development, and good eyesight.
- Pumpkin is rich in dietary fiber, which helps the digestive system by encouraging regular bowel motions and supporting gut health.

Health Benefits

1. **Eye Health**: Pumpkin's high Good for your eyes, thanks to the beta-carotene and vitamin A in it. In addition to being essential for healthy eyes, these nutrients may ward against age-related macular degeneration and night blindness.
2. **Immune System Support**: The vitamin A derived from beta-carotene, along with vitamin C in pumpkins, increases the body's resistance to disease and infection by strengthening the immune system.

3. Pumpkin's fiber aids digestion by increasing stool volume and encouraging regular bowel movements, which in turn helps avoid constipation.

Snake Gourd (Chichinda)

Snake gourd is an excellent source of nutrients and has many positive effects on health. I have a detailed look at its nutritional content and health benefits:

Nutritional Content

Vitamins: Snake gourd is an excellent source of vitamin A and vitamin C, which are necessary for healthy skin, eyes, and immune system.

Fibre: Packed with dietary fiber, which supports healthy digestion and encourages regular bowel movements.

Health Benefits

1. **Digestive Health**: The high fiber content of snake gourd aids digestion by reducing constipation and increasing stool volume.
2. **Weight control:** By increasing fullness and decreasing calorie intake, snake gourd is great for weight control since it is low in calories and rich in water content.
3. Snake gourd helps the immune system fight off infections and diseases since it is rich in vitamins A and C more effectively.

Ridge Gourd (Tori)

Ridge gourd is another nutritious vegetable with various health benefits:

Nutritional Content

Vitamins and Minerals: Rich in dietary fiber, vitamin C, and iron. Some of the many body processes that these nutrients aid with include digestion and immune system support.

Health Benefits

1. **Digestive Health**: Ridge gourd's high fiber content helps with digestion by encouraging regular bowel movements and bolstering gut health.
2. The immune system is bolstered by the vitamin C found in ridge gourd, which increases the formation of white blood cells.
3. **Iron Content**: Provides iron, essential for producing hemoglobin and maintaining healthy blood cells.

Mustard Greens (Sarson)

Nutritional Content:

Vitamins: Vitamins A, C, and K abound in mustard greens. Blood coagulation and bone health are both greatly aided by vitamin K, while the antioxidant properties of vitamins A and C ensure that support immune function and skin health.

Antioxidants: Antioxidants like beta-carotene and flavonoids found in them help ward against oxidative damage and inflammation.

Health Benefits:

Bone Health: The high vitamin K content in mustard greens helps maintain bone mineralization and calcium absorption, which in turn lowers the incidence of fractures and increases bone density.

Mustard greens' antioxidants, including beta-carotene and vitamin C, may decrease inflammation and may lessen the likelihood of chronic inflammatory illnesses. This is known as their anti-inflammatory properties.

Heart Health: Studies have shown that mustard greens may help keep your heart healthy. Compounds in these foods aid in the digestion process by binding bile acids, which in turn may reduce cholesterol levels and promote heart health

Coriander (Dhania)

Nutritional Content:

Vitamins: Coriander contains antioxidants, vitamin K, and vitamin C. In contrast to vitamin K's central role in blood clotting and bone health, vitamin C is vital for immune function and skin health.

One benefit of coriander is the abundance of antioxidants it contains. These compounds shield cells from harmful oxidative stress and inflammation.

Health Benefits:

Digestive Health: Coriander aids digestion by stimulating enzymatic digestion, which aids in food breakdown and enhances nutritional absorption. If you're experiencing indigestion or gas, this may assist.

Healthy Skin: Improved skin health is a result of vitamin C and the antioxidants in coriander, which help to decrease free radical damage and boost collagen synthesis, which keeps the skin firm and youthful.

Other Benefits: Coriander may also provide antimicrobial benefits for people with diabetes because to its anti-inflammatory and anti-infective characteristics and its link to reduced blood sugar levels.

Curry Leaves:

Nutritional Content:

- **Vitamins**: You may get a lot of vitamin A, B, C, and E from curry leaves. Having healthy skin, eyes, and an immune system are just a few of the many biological processes that rely on these vitamins. The immune system and skin health are supported by vitamin C, while eyesight is especially helped by vitamin A.
- **Additional Nutrients**: Curry leaves also contain essential nutrients like calcium, iron, and various antioxidants.

Health Benefits:

1. **Hair Health**: The hair-health advantages of curry leaves are well-known. Their actions include fortifying hair follicles, increasing hair growth, and decreasing hair loss. In addition to nourishing the scalp, the antifungal qualities of the leaves make them useful for avoiding dandruff.

2. Curry leaves aid digestion by increasing the activity of digestive enzymes and facilitating the breakdown of fats. They are known to help alleviate digestive issues like indigestion and diarrhea.
3. **Antioxidant Properties**: The antioxidants in curry leaves reduce the likelihood of developing chronic illnesses by shielding cells from oxidative stress and free radical damage.

Drumstick (Moringa)

Nutritional Content:

- **Vitamins**: Drumsticks are a good source of the vitamins A, C, and E that the body needs for a number of processes.
- Vitamins A, C, and E are essential for proper eyesight and immunological function, healthy skin, and strong immune systems, respectively protects cells from oxidative damage.
- **Calcium**: Moringa includes calcium, an essential mineral for healthy teeth and bones. Neuronal signaling and muscular function are both aided by it.

Health Benefits:

1. **Boosts Immunity**: In order to fight off infections, your immune system needs white blood cells, and the abundance of vitamins A and C in moringa helps produce more of them.
2. **Promotes Strong Bones**: The high levels of calcium and phosphorus found in moringa are essential for strong bones. Conditions like osteoporosis may be prevented with their aid in bone mineralization.
3. **Anti-inflammatory and Antioxidant Properties:** Moringa's antioxidants mitigate inflammation and shield cells from

oxidative stress, hence decreasing the likelihood of developing chronic illnesses.

Amaranth Leaves (Chaulai)
Nutritional Content:

- **Vitamins**: Amaranth leaves are high in vitamins A and C. Vitamin A is necessary for good eyesight and immunological function, while vitamin C is an effective antioxidant that shields cells from harm and strengthens the immune system.
- These leaves are a good source of iron, a mineral necessary for the body to make hemoglobin, the protein responsible for transporting oxygen throughout the body, and helps prevent anemia.

Health Benefits:

1. **Eye Health**: To keep your eyes healthy and your eyesight sharp, eat amaranth leaves. They are rich in vitamin A, which is essential for warding off night blindness. To keep the retina healthy and the eyes functioning properly, it is crucial to consume enough vitamin A.
2. They help with digestion by encouraging regular bowel movements and warding off constipation thanks to the high fiber content of amaranth leaves. Fiber promotes regular bowel movements by increasing stool volume.
3. amaranth leaves have antioxidant qualities that aid in inflammation reduction and oxidative stress protection for the body. As a result, the likelihood of chronic diseases and support overall health

Swiss chard

Nutritional Content:

- **Vitamins**: Swiss Vitamins K, A, and C are abundant in chard. Vitamins A and C are potent antioxidants; vitamin K is necessary for healthy blood coagulation and bones; vitamin A aids eyesight and the immune system; and vitamin C boosts immune health and skin integrity.
- **Magnesium**: This mineral helps the body use energy, maintains healthy bones, and works the muscles and nerves.

Health Benefits:

1. **Bone Health**: Swiss chard supports bone health primarily due to it aids in the process of bone mineralization and has a high concentration of vitamin K, maintain bone density. The presence of magnesium and calcium further contributes to strengthening bones.
2. **Reduces Inflammation**: Swiss chard is rich in antioxidants and vitamins, especially A and C, which aid reduce inflammation throughout the body. Vitamin K also contributes to managing inflammation, which could help with aches and pains like arthritis.
3. Swiss chard is good for your heart since it has heart-healthy minerals and a lot of fiber, which assist control your blood pressure and cholesterol.

Green Beans

Nutritional Content:

Vitamins: Green beans are rich in K, A, and C vitamins. Vitamins A, C, and K are crucial for many bodily functions, including vision, immunity, skin, and blood clotting and bone health, respectively. Vitamin C is an effective antioxidant that helps the immune system and promotes healthy skin.

1. **Fiber**: They include a lot of dietary fiber, which helps with digestion and keeps cholesterol levels in check, which is beneficial for your heart.

Health Advantages:

1. Green beans' high fiber content aids in lowering levels of bad cholesterol (LDL), which in turn lowers the risk of heart disease. Green beans may also aid with blood pressure regulation and cardiovascular health due to the folate and potassium they contain.
2. they're great for your bones since green beans are full of vitamin K. Increased bone strength and decreased fracture risk are both outcomes of vitamin K's role in modifying proteins that make up the bone matrix.
3. **Anti-inflammatory Benefits**: Vitamin C and other antioxidants found in green beans aid reduce inflammation and oxidative stress, which can lower the risk of chronic diseases

Hence vegetables are an essential component of a healthy diet, providing a wide range of vital nutrients such as vitamins, minerals, fiber, and antioxidants. These nutrients support various bodily functions, including immune function, bone health, digestion, and cardiovascular health. By incorporating a diverse array of vegetables like mustard greens, coriander, curry leaves, drumstick, amaranth leaves, Swiss chard, and green beans into your meals, you can enjoy both the flavorful diversity and the numerous health benefits they offer. Embracing a diet rich in vegetables contributes to overall well-being and helps prevent chronic diseases, making them a cornerstone of a balanced, nutritious lifestyle

18

EXPLORING THE HEALING POWER OF HERBS

𝒫lants and plant components that have flavor, scent, or therapeutic value are called herbs. Their traditional medicinal usage dates back centuries to treat various ailments. Below is a detailed explanation of the health benefits of few herbs

Aloe Vera:

The therapeutic qualities of the succulent plant species Aloe Vera have been known for generations. Its leaf gel is an excellent source of several beneficial chemicals, such as:

1. The nutritional content of aloe vera includes choline, folic acid, vitamins A, C, and E, and vitamin B12. A healthy immune system, glowing skin, and good health are all benefits of these vitamins.

2. **Enzymes**: This plant has a number of enzymes that help break down fats and proteins and may even lower inflammatory levels.
3. **Minerals**: It contains minerals including iron, sodium, potassium, chromium, selenium, magnesium, zinc, and calcium essential for various bodily functions.
4. **Sugars**: Aloe Vera contains complex carbohydrates, including acemannan and glucomannan, which have been researched for the possible advantages to health, including immune system support.
5. **Lignin**: This natural substance helps the body absorb the nutrients from Aloe Vera more effectively.
6. **Saponins**: These are natural cleansing agents that can help with detoxification and have antibacterial properties.
7. **Salicylic Acids**: These are useful for treating skin disorders like acne because of their antibacterial and anti-inflammatory characteristics.
8. Among the 22 amino acids needed by the human body, 20 are found in aloe vera. This includes all eight essential amino acids that we cannot synthesize ourselves.

Health Benefits

➢ **Wound Healing**: Aloe Vera Because of its anti-inflammatory characteristics and its capacity to promote skin development and regeneration, it helps hasten the healing of wounds, small burns, and skin injuries.
➢ A more supple and hydrated skin, less wrinkles, and relief from skin problems like eczema and psoriasis are all benefits of using Aloe Vera on a regular basis.

➢ Arthritis and inflammatory skin disorders are two examples of conditions that might benefit from Aloe Vera's anti-inflammatory properties, which it exhibits both topically and orally.

Ginseng:

Ginseng is a popular herbal supplement that originated in Asia and has a long history of use in traditional medicine there. Its adaptogenic qualities make it a popular choice for those looking to strengthen their immune systems. I have included some important aspects here points about ginseng and its active components:

Active Components

1. **Ginsenosides**: These are the primary active compounds in ginseng, responsible for many of its health benefits. Ginsenosides are triterpene saponins that are known to have neuroprotective, antioxidant, and anti-inflammatory properties.
2. **Gintonin**: This is another active component found in ginseng, particularly in its root. Gintonin has been shown to have neuroprotective properties and may help in the treatment of neurodegenerative diseases.

Health Benefits

1. **Energy Boost**: Ginseng is often used to enhance physical and mental energy. Because of its ability to lessen weariness and increase stamina, it has become a popular supplement among athletes and individuals seeking a natural energy boost.

2. **Stress Reduction**: Ginseng has characteristics that promote adaptability, allowing the body to better handle stressful situations. It has the potential to lower cortisol and other stress hormone levels, which in turn may improve mood and physical health.
3. **Enhancement of Cognitive Function**: Research indicates that ginseng may promote better cognitive function, which encompasses memory, concentration, and overall mental performance. This is partly due to the neuroprotective effects of ginsenosides and gintonin.
4. **Anti-inflammatory Properties**: Ginseng's Anti-inflammatory effects have the ability to decrease systemic inflammation, which is advantageous for a range of medical problems, such as inflammatory illnesses like arthritis.

Garlic:

Garlic (Allium sativum) is a widely used culinary herb that also boasts Garlic has a plethora of health advantages, mostly because of the allicin it contains. Crushing or chopping garlic releases an enzyme called alliinase, which interacts with the amino acid alliin to generate allicin, a sulfur-containing chemical. The many ways in which garlic helps the heart, the immune system, and the environment (including via its antibacterial and antioxidant properties) are outlined here:

1. **Heart Health**
   Researchers have looked into garlic's effects on cardiovascular health in great detail. The allicin in it may help relax the blood arteries, which in turn lowers blood pressure.

Reduced risk of atherosclerosis is one benefit of consuming garlic, which lowers levels of both total and LDL (bad) cholesterol.

Because of its antiplatelet characteristics, allicin may lessen the likelihood of blood clot formation and, by extension, the likelihood of cardiovascular events like heart attacks and strokes.

Boost Blood Flow: Garlic may improve circulation by lowering inflammation and increasing blood flow can enhance overall cardiovascular health.

2. **Infectious Agents**

A stronger immune system is one of garlic's well-known benefits. Allicin and other garlic components may boost the activity of immune cells like macrophages and T cells, which are vital for fighting off infections. This enhances immune cell function.

➤ **Decrease Inflammation**: The immune response may be modulated by garlic's anti-inflammatory properties, stopping excessive inflammation that can lead to chronic diseases.

➤ **Fight Infections:** When it comes to fighting germs, viruses, and fungus, garlic is your best bet. It may aid the immune system in its battle against typical illnesses.

➤ **Antimicrobial Effects**

➤ Garlic's antimicrobial properties are well-documented:

➤ **Bacterial Infections:** Allicin has shown antibacterial activity against a range of microorganisms, including Helicobacter pylori, Staphylococcus aureus, and Escherichia coli.

- **Infections caused by viruses:** research indicates that garlic may prevent the spread of some viruses, such as the flu virus and even HIV.
- **Fungal Infections:** Garlic can also combat fungal infections; therefore, it may be used as a helpful natural treatment for yeast infections and athlete's foot

4. **Antioxidant Effects**

   Garlic is a potent antioxidant, which means by reducing free radical damage and oxidative stress, it may aid in protecting the body. Because it neutralizes free radicals, garlic helps protect cells from harm, including DNA damage and cancer-causing mutations.

Garlic's anti-oxidant properties make it a useful tool in the fight against oxidative stress, a risk factor for a host of chronic illnesses (such as cardiovascular disease and neurological problems).

Supporting the body's natural detoxification processes, garlic aids in the elimination of toxic substances toxins and chemicals.

The Tiger Milk Mushroom:

The Tiger Milk Mushroom, scientifically known as Lignosus rhinocerotis, is a highly valued classic medicinal fungus that has a long and storied history of usage, especially in Southeast Asian medicine. Its distinctive nutritional profile and bioactive components are responsible for its well-deserved reputation for powerful health benefits.

Nutritional Composition

The Tiger Milk Mushroom is rich in various nutrients and bioactive compounds which help explain why it's good for you. A few examples include:

- **Polysaccharides**: Renown for the immune-enhancing benefits they provide.
- **Triterpenoids**: Compounds with anti-inflammatory and antioxidant effects.
- **Other Bioactive Compounds**: Such as ergosterol, which is associated with proper immunological function and the stability of cell membranes.

Health Benefits

The Tiger Milk Mushroom offers many different kinds of health advantages, which fall into a few main categories:

1. **Immune System Support**:
   Enhances immune function by boosting resilience in the face of illness and infection. Let me clarify supported by its polysaccharide content, which is known to stimulate immune responses.
2. **Respiratory Health**:
   Helps promote better respiratory health by decreasing airway and lung inflammation. This is particularly effective in relieving coughs, improving breathing, and supporting healthy mucus production, which can help clear the airway.
3. **Anti-inflammatory Properties**:
   Reduces systemic inflammation, which may provide relief for a range of inflammatory conditions including arthritis and

asthma. The triterpenoids in the mushroom are primarily responsible for these anti-inflammatory effects.

4. **Antioxidant Action**:
Protects the body from free radical neutralization alleviates oxidative stress. The general health of cells is aided by this antioxidant action and can help prevent damage to cells and tissues.

5. **Cognitive Support**:
May support brain health and cognitive function. Similar to lion's mane mushroom, it is believed to have neuroprotective properties that can enhance brain function and memory.

6. **Anticancer Properties**:
Tiger Milk Mushroom may have anticancer benefits, according to certain studies. However, more study is required to completely understand how it prevents and treats cancer.

7. **Detoxification**:
Helps in cleansing and detoxifying the lungs, which can be beneficial for smokers and those with respiratory issues

Monascus

Monascus, commonly known as red yeast rice, is a fermented product of rice that has been grown with the red yeast Monascus purpureus. This unique substance has been used in Chinese cuisine and as a medicinal food for centuries, primarily for its health benefits.

Health Benefits of Monascus

1. **Cholesterol Management**: Monascus is particularly noted for its capacity to reduce cholesterol levels. It contains compounds

like monacolins, which are similar to statins and can effectively reduce total cholesterol and low-density lipoprotein (LDL) cholesterol levels, thereby reducing the risk of cardiovascular diseases.

2. **Cardiovascular Health**: By lowering cholesterol, Monascus also helps in improving cardiovascular health. It lowers the danger of cardiovascular disease, which includes heart attacks and strokes.
3. **Diabetes Management**: Monascus has been shown to have beneficial effects on diabetes. Through modulating glucose metabolism, it may aid in glucose management and the prevention of diabetes.
4. **Anti-inflammatory Properties:** Monascus contains chemicals, such monacolins, that have the ability to reduce inflammation in the body. This may have positive effects on general health.
5. **Cancer Prevention:** Monascus has been linked to a reduced risk of cancer in some research preventing cancer. It contains compounds that can inhibit the growth of cancer cells and reduce the risk of certain types of cancer.

Roselle

Roselle, also known as Hibiscus sabdariffa, is a plant with a rich history of use in traditional medicine and is valued for its nutritional and medicinal properties. Here are the key components and health benefits of Roselle based on the provided references:

Content

1. **Vitamin C**: The immune system and skin both rely on vitamin C, which roselle provides in plenty. Consuming 100 grams of raw Roselle offers 12 mg of vitamin C.
2. **Calcium and Iron**: Additionally, it contains iron and calcium, two elements crucial to strong bones and red blood cell production, respectively. 100 grams of raw Roselle contains 215 mg of calcium and 1.48 mg of iron.
3. **Polyphenols**: The aqueous extract of Roselle is rich in several polyphenols; they are well-known for the anti-inflammatory and antioxidant effects they have.
4. Antioxidants like flavonoids and anthocyanins lower cholesterol and blood pressure and improve cardiovascular health.

Health Benefits

1. **Immune System Support**: Roselle guards against common infections by bolstering the immune system with its high vitamin C concentration.
2. **Blood Pressure Regulation**: Roselle has been shown to have antihypertensive properties, helping to reduce hypertension and control hypertension.
3. **Cholesterol Management**: When used for cardiac rehabilitation, it helps dysfunction by removing toxic and unwanted cholesterol from the body, thus helping to lower cholesterol levels.
4. **Liver Wellness:** Roselle has a long history of use in traditional medicine as a means to prevent liver problems and reduce the risk of liver damage.

5. **Anti-inflammatory Effects**: The polyphenols and antioxidants in Roselle contribute to it helps manage a range of inflammatory diseases due to its anti-inflammatory effects.
6. Roselle's anti-diabetic properties have been studied, and it has shown promise in controlling blood sugar levels, which might help with diabetes management.
7. Roselle may have anticancer qualities, according to certain studies; nevertheless, more study is required to completely understand its impact on cancer prevention and therapy.

Wild Betel

Wild Betel, Native to South and Southeast Asia, this plant has a long history of medicinal usage under its scientific name, Piper betle. Its distinctive taste and many health advantages have made it famous. The following are the main features and health advantages of Wild Betel:

Content

1. **Alkaloids**: Wild Betel contains several members of the alkaloid class, including the stimulant arecoline.
2. **Flavonoids**: These antioxidants help in reducing inflammation and oxidative stress.
3. **Phenolic Compounds**: These chemicals help make the plant anti-inflammatory and antioxidant.
4. **Minerals and Vitamins:** Wild betel contains minerals like iron and calcium and vitamins like vitamin C.

Health Benefits

1. **Oral Health**: Chewing Wild Betel leaves is traditionally believed to help in maintaining oral hygiene and freshening breath.
2. **Digestive Health**: Its digestive and constipation-relieving properties are well-known. The stimulant properties of arecoline can help in increasing gut motility.
3. **Anti-inflammatory Effects**: The flavonoids and phenolic compounds in Wild Betel help in reducing inflammation, that may help in the management of a range of inflammatory disorders.
4. **Wild Betel's Antioxidant Properties:** Wild Betel's antioxidants shield cells from cellular damage and oxidative stress.
5. **Supporting the Immune System:** Wild Betel's vitamin C concentration aids in enhancing the immune system, shielding the body from frequent infections.
6. Wild betel has a long history of traditional usage in the treatment of coughs, bronchitis, and other respiratory illnesses.
7. **The Potential Benefits to Cardiovascular Health:** Research indicates that Wild Betel might potentially have benefits, although more research is needed to fully understand its effects on heart health.

Spirulina

Spirulina, a type of blue-green algae, is renowned for its nutritional profile and health benefits. Here are the key components and health benefits of Spirulina:

Nutritional Components

1. **Protein**: Vegans and vegetarians may benefit greatly from spirulina as a protein supplement since it contains all the important amino acids.
2. **Vitamins**: It's an excellent way to get your daily dose of vitamins A, B complex, and K.
3. Spirulina, a mineral contains minerals like iron, magnesium, calcium, and potassium.
4. **Fatty Acids**: It includes both needed fatty acids for healthy health, including *omega-3 and omega-6.*
5. **Phycocyanin**: This is the main active compound in spirulina, well-known for its ability to reduce inflammation and act as an antioxidant.

Health Benefits

1. **Antioxidant Properties**: Spirulina is an excellent source of antioxidants, which defend cells from oxidative stress and free radical damage.
2. **Heart Health**: It may help in lowering cholesterol and triglyceride levels, which can support heart health.
3. **Blood Pressure Regulation**: Spirulina may boost NO production, which aids in vasodilation and reduces blood pressure.
4. **Weight Management:** Spirulina may help with weight reduction by blocking the small intestine's ability to absorb fat, according to some research.
5. **Digestive Health:** It has the potential to improve digestive health by encouraging the development of good bacteria.

6. **Support for the Immune System:** Research has shown that spirulina may enhance the immune system's function by promoting the synthesis of antibodies and infection-fighting proteins.
7. **Anti-inflammatory Effects**: Reduced inflammation is one of the benefits of spirulina's antioxidants, which is beneficial for managing various inflammatory conditions.
8. **Skin Health**: Essential nutrients and antioxidants included in spirulina may aid in skin health improvement antioxidants

Cordyceps

Cordyceps, a type of fungus, includes a number of bioactive components that help explain its beneficial effects on health. The main active components include:

1. **Cordycepin**: This is a nucleoside analog that has been the subject of research due to its possible anti-inflammatory effects and other health benefits conditions such as asthma, rheumatoid arthritis, Parkinson's disease, hepatitis, and more.
2. **Adenosine**: This compound is known for its role in improving exercise performance and enhancing the body's use of oxygen.
3. **Polysaccharides**: These believed to possess anti-inflammatory and antioxidant characteristics, are important water-soluble components of the fungus.
4. **Other Nutrients**: Cordyceps also contains vitamins (like B vitamins and vitamin K), mineral salts (sodium, potassium, calcium, magnesium, iron, zinc, and selenium) and lysine, threonine, and proline, among other necessary amino acids.

Health Benefits of Cordyceps

Cordyceps has several positive effects on health, including as:

1. **Improved Athletic Performance**: Cordyceps may enhance exercise performance by improving the body's use of oxygen, which can delay fatigue.
2. **Heart Health**: It has the potential to control heart rate and enhance blood cholesterol levels, which is beneficial for heart health.
3. **Anti-inflammatory Effects**: Cordycepin, a key component, has been found to regulate certain pathways that are implicated in inflammation, which might provide a defense against inflammatory disorders that persist over time.
4. Cordyceps may have anti-aging properties, according to some research process by increasing antioxidant levels and improving memory and sexual function in aged mice.
5. **Anti-tumor Effects**: Research indicates that cordyceps may impede the proliferation of certain cancer cells and perhaps alleviate leukopenia, a side effect of cancer therapy.
6. **Managing Diabetes:** It has the potential to assist in controlling blood sugar levels and protect against nerve damage caused by diabetes.
7. **Immune System Support**: Cordyceps the immune system by boosting the activity and generation of different types of immune cells; it may also aid the body in adapting to stress and exhaustion; thus, it is classified as an adaptogen.

Agaricus Blazei Murill

Agaricus Blazei Murill, commonly known as the Royal Sun Agaric or Brazilian mushroom, has a number of bioactive ingredients that make it beneficial to health. Here are the key ingredients:

1. **Polysaccharides**: These are immunomodulating polysaccharides, particularly β-glucans, They are well-known for the immune-boosting effects they provide.
2. **Nucleic Acids:** Nucleic acids play an important role in many physiological functions and might be one reason why the mushroom.
3. **Vitamins and Minerals**: Agaricus Blazei Murill contains essential vitamins like essential elements including magnesium and calcium, as well as vitamin B2.

Health Benefits of Agaricus Blazei Murill

Agaricus Blazei Murill provides several health advantages, such as:

1. **Immune System Support**: Its immune-stimulatory effect has made it famous and has the potential to in boosting the immune system and fighting infections .
2. **Anti-cancer Properties**: The mushroom has been studied for its potential in inhibiting tumor growth and preventing cancer .
3. **Anti-inflammatory Effects**: Agaricus Blazei Murill may help in reducing inflammation, which may help alleviate a range of inflammatory illnesses.
4. **Effects on Diabetes**: It aids in lowering insulin resistance and managing type 2 diabetes .
5. **Anti-allergic Properties**: The mushroom may help in reducing allergic reactions and asthma symptoms

6. **Cardiovascular Health**: It may help in improving improve blood circulation and lower cholesterol levels, which is good for the heart.
7. **Liver Health**: Agaricus Blazei Murill may support liver health and protect against liver damage .
8. **Antioxidant Properties**: The mushroom includes protective antioxidants that the body needs from oxidative stress and cellular damage

Ganoderma lucidum

Ganoderma lucidum, commonly known as Reishi or Lingzhi, has a number of bioactive ingredients that make it beneficial to health. Here are the key parts:

1. **Polysaccharides**: These enhance the body's defensive systems and are recognized for their immune-boosting qualities.
2. **Triterpenes:** These substances are rich in antioxidant and anti-inflammatory characteristics; they include beneficial for managing various health conditions.
3. **Beta-glucans**: Found in the caps and stems of the mushroom, beta-glucans are known for their immune-modulating effects.
4. **Adenosine**: This compound is involved in improving energy levels and enhancing the body's use of oxygen.
5. **Germanium**: An effective antioxidant that promotes better cellular oxygenation and aids in the body's detoxification processes.
6. The sixth point is the presence of proteins and enzymes, which help the mushroom by supporting various physiological functions.

Health Benefits of Ganoderma lucidum

Ganoderma Lucidum has several health advantages, such as:

1. **Immune System Support**: It enhances strengthens the immune system, which in turn helps the body fight off illnesses and infections.
2. **Anti-inflammatory Effects**: The triterpenes and polysaccharides in Ganoderma lucidum help in reducing inflammation, which may help alleviate a range of inflammatory disorders.
3. **Antioxidant Properties**: The antioxidants it contains help keep harmful free radicals and cell damage at bay.
4. Ganoderma lucidum, a potential regulator of blood pressure and cholesterol levels, may contribute to better cardiovascular health.
5. **Detoxification**: The organic germanium in Ganoderma lucidum aids in detoxifying the body and improving cellular oxygenation.
6. **Weight Management**: It may help in managing weight by boosting metabolism and aiding in fat burning.
7. **Nervous System Health**: Ganoderma lucidum enhances attention and focus, aids in stress and anxiety reduction, and supports overall nervous system health

Valeriana jatamansi

Valeriana jatamansi, commonly known as Indian Valerian, is a perennial medicinal herb used in traditional and modern medicine. The rhizome of this plant contains several bioactive compounds that contribute to its health benefits. The main components include:

1. **Valepotriates**: These are major active components found in the roots and rhizomes of Valeriana jatamansi, which are used in folk medicine in Asia.
2. **Iridoid Glycosides**: These are also significant components of Valeriana jatamansi, known for their medicinal properties.
3. **Essential Oils**: The essential oils of Valeriana jatamansi include compounds like Patchoulic alcohol, could help make its medicinal benefits known.

Health Benefits of Valeriana jatamansi Rhizome

Valeriana There are many health advantages associated with jatamansi rhizome, including as:

1. **Sleep Aid**: It is commonly used to treat insomnia and improve sleep quality, which can help reduce anxiety and depression.
2. **Anti-inflammatory Effects**: The rhizome extract has been shown to reduce inflammation in rats, indicating its potential in managing inflammatory conditions.
3. **Neurological Health**: Valeriana jatamansi is used in the treatment of neuronal problems, suggesting its potential in neurological health.
4. **Antispasmodic Properties**: The rhizome is used as a raw tonic and antispasmodic in Ayurvedic medicine, which can help in treating conditions like hysteria, convulsions, and epilepsy.
5. **Antioxidant Properties**: The essential oils of Valeriana jatamansi exhibit antioxidant activity, which can help in protecting the body from oxidative stress

Omega-3 fatty acids

Omega-3 fatty acids, found in fish oil and flaxseeds, are essential nutrients that play a crucial role in various bodily functions, particularly in supporting heart health, reducing inflammation, and promoting brain health.

Heart Health

Omega-3 fatty acids, particularly EPA and DHA, have been extensively studied for their benefits in cardiovascular health. They can help lower triglyceride levels, reduce inflammation, and improve blood flow, which are all factors that contribute to a reduced risk of heart disease and stroke. A systematic review and meta-analysis found that omega-3 fatty acids were associated with reduced cardiovascular mortality and other outcomes. Additionally, omega-3 supplements have been linked to a lower risk of heart attack, coronary heart disease, and total heart disease.

Inflammation Reduction

Omega-3 fatty acids are known for their anti-inflammatory properties. They can help regulate the inflammatory response by influencing the production of inflammatory proteins. This is particularly beneficial in conditions like rheumatoid arthritis and inflammatory bowel disease, where omega-3 supplements have been shown to reduce pain and improve symptoms.

Brain Health

Omega-3 fatty acids are crucial for brain development and function. DHA, a type of omega-3, is a major structural component of the brain and is essential for cognitive function and memory. Studies have shown that omega-3 supplementation can help protect against cognitive decline and promote healthy brain functioning in both older and younger populations. Omega-3 fatty acids are also important for brain development in infants and may help reduce symptoms of depression and anxiety.

Sources of Omega-3 Fatty Acids

- **Fish Oil**: The best omega-3 fatty acids for cardiovascular and neurological health are EPA and DHA, which are abundant in this oil.
- The body can convert ALA, which is found in flaxseeds, into EPA and DHA, but at a very low rate.
- The Southeast Asian tropical fruit Garcinia Cambogia has gained popularity due to its purported weight loss and hunger suppressant properties.

Garcinia Cambogia

Garcinia Cambogia contains Hydroxycitric Acid (HCA), the active ingredient, and it is believed to contribute to its health benefits.

Compounds in Garcinia Cambogia

The primary active compound in Garcinia Cambogia is Hydroxycitric Acid (HCA). HCA is extracted from the rind of the fruit and is thought to have several effects that contribute to weight loss and appetite reduction:

1. **Inhibition of Citrate Lyase**: The enzyme citrate lyase is involved in the the process that HCA is thought to block synthesis of fatty acids. By blocking this enzyme, HCA may

reduce the conversion of carbohydrates into fat, potentially leading to reduced fat storage.
2. **Increased Serotonin Levels**: HCA may also raise brain serotonin levels. Serotonin is a neurotransmitter that can influence appetite and mood. Higher serotonin levels are associated with reduced appetite and a feeling of satiety, which can lead to decreased food intake.

Health Benefits of Garcinia Cambogia

Garcinia Cambogia is commonly marketed for its potential to aid in weight loss and appetite control. Here are some of the health benefits associated with Garcinia Cambogia:

1. **Weight Loss**: Garcinia Cambogia is often used as it may help with weight reduction if used properly. Possible benefits include less hunger and fatter burning, which might lead to overall weight loss.
2. **Appetite Control**: HCA is thought to reduce appetite by increasing serotonin levels, it may aid in managing food consumption and cutting down on calories generally.
3. Cholesterol and Blood Fat Levels: Garcinia Cambogia may have a role in reducing levels of cholesterol and blood fat, which are crucial for cardiovascular health, according to some research.
4. Garcinia Cambogia may also aid with mood enhancement by raising serotonin levels mood and reduce stress-related eating

Ginkgo Biloba

Ginkgo Biloba, one of the oldest living tree species, has been used in traditional Chinese medicine for centuries. It is renowned for its potential health benefits, particularly in enhancing memory and cognitive function, as well as improving circulation. The active compounds in Ginkgo Biloba are flavonoids and terpenoids, which contribute to its therapeutic effects.

Active Compounds

1. **Flavonoids**: These are a group of plant-based substances that neutralize free radicals and hence help the body fight it. There are flavonoids in Ginkgo Biloba, such kaempferol and quercetin, which can lower inflammation and protect neurons from damage.
2. **Terpenoids**: These are another group of compounds found in Ginkgo Biloba, including ginkgolides and bilobalide. Terpenoids have been shown to have neuroprotective properties, improve blood flow, and inhibit platelet-activating factor (PAF), which is involved in inflammation and blood clotting.

Health Benefits

1. **Enhancing Memory and Cognitive Function**: Ginkgo Biloba is often used help enhance mental acuity and memory. Terpenoids' neuroprotective effects and flavonoids' antioxidant capabilities may shield the brain against oxidative stress and neurodegenerative illnesses. Another possible mechanism by which Ginkgo Biloba improves cognitive performance is via increasing cerebral blood flow.
2. **Improving Circulation**: The terpenoids in Ginkgo Biloba, particularly ginkgolides, can inhibit PAF, which is involved in inflammation and blood clotting. This can help improve

circulation by reducing the stickiness of platelets and preventing blood clots. Improved circulation can also benefit the brain, leading to better cognitive function.

Mechanism of Action

1. **Antioxidant Effects**: The flavonoids in Ginkgo Biloba act as antioxidants, preventing oxidative stress on cells and scavenging free radicals. This is particularly beneficial for brain cells, which are vulnerable to oxidative stress.
2. **Neuroprotection**: Terpenoids, such as bilobalide, have been shown to protect neurons from damage. They may aid in keeping neuronal membranes intact, which is necessary for neuronal survival.
3. **Vasodilation**: Because of its ability to widen blood vessels, Ginkgo Biloba improves blood flow to many parts of the body, including the brain. A rise in cerebral blood flow has the potential to improve mental performance and reduce the risk of cardiovascular diseases.

Fenugreek

Fenugreek is an herb with several notable health benefits, including supporting digestion, regulating blood sugar, and possessing anti-inflammatory properties. Here's a detailed look at these benefits:

1. **Supports Digestion**: Fenugreek can aid in digestion by acting as a natural fiber source. It helps in softening stools and may relieve constipation, enhancing overall gut wellness. The soluble fiber in fenugreek seeds may help with gastrointestinal

issues like bloating and gas by reducing the rate at which carbs are digested and absorbed.
2. Fenugreek is useful for diabetics and those at risk of getting diabetes since it regulates blood sugar levels. It may help reduce blood sugar levels by inhibiting the stomach's ability to absorb sugar and by increasing insulin production. Research indicates that fenugreek may enhance insulin sensitivity and glucose tolerance.
3. Fenugreek may be useful in reducing inflammation since it contains chemicals with anti-inflammatory properties. Arthritis and other inflammatory illnesses may benefit greatly from this. Reduce your risk of chronic inflammatory diseases with the help of fenugreek's anti-inflammatory characteristics.

Liquorice

Liquorice (Glycyrrhiza glabra) is a plant has a long history of usage in alternative medicine, most notably in Ayurvedic and Chinese medicine. Its active ingredient is mostly responsible for its famed sweet flavor and many health advantages compound glycyrrhizin.

Active Compound: Glycyrrhizin

Glycyrrhizin is a triterpenoid saponin that is primarily reason why licorice is good for you. In addition to strengthening the immune system, it offers powerful anti-inflammatory and antioxidant effects.

Health Benefits

1. **Anti-inflammatory Properties**: Glycyrrhizin may aid in reducing inflammation in the body because to its significant anti-inflammatory actions. Conditions include inflammatory disorders, ulcerative colitis, and arthritis may benefit from this.
2. **Immune-Boosting Effects**: Liquorice can help enhance immune function by modulating immune cell function. A higher level of the infection-fighting cytokines, such as interferons, may be produced.
3. **Antiviral Properties**: Research has shown that lycyrrhizin may inhibit the growth of many viruses, including HIV, herpes simplex, and hepatitis C. In addition to protecting cells from viral harm, it may also suppress viral replication.
4. **Liquorice's Adaptogenic Properties:** The body may use licorice, which is an adaptogen, to better withstand stress. It has the potential to improve mood and control the body's reaction to stress.
5. **Digestive Health**: Liquorice can help soothe the gastrointestinal tract and is often used to treat conditions such as gastric ulcers and indigestion. It can help reduce inflammation and protect the mucous membranes of the stomach.

Lycium barbarum

Lycium barbarum, commonly known as Goji berries, is a fruit that has been used in traditional Chinese medicine for centuries. These small, red berries are packed with vitamins, minerals, and antioxidants, making them a nutritious addition to the diet. Here's a detailed look at their health benefits:

Nutritional Profile

Goji berries are rich in various nutrients, including:

- **Vitamins**: Rich in beta-carotene, a kind of vitamin A, as well as vitamin C and magnesium (riboflavin).
- **Minerals**: Include vital elements like selenium, calcium, iron, and zinc.
- **Antioxidants**: Rich in antioxidants like carotenoids and polysaccharides.

Health Benefits

1. **Eye Health**: Goji berries are known for their potential to support eye health. They contain zeaxanthin, a carotenoid that has positive effects on eye health and might provide protection against cataracts and age-related macular degeneration (AMD).
2. Goji berries may improve immunological function because to their high vitamin C content. White blood cells are vital for fighting off infections, and vitamin C is required for their formation.
3. **Anti-Aging Benefits**: The antioxidants in Goji berries may aid in preventing oxidative stress, a key factor in the aging process. Free radicals may cause harm to cells, although antioxidants can counteract this.
4. **Skin Health:** Goji berries' vitamin and antioxidant content may aid skin health by shielding it from harmful environmental contaminants and ultraviolet light.
5. Goji berries may have actions that protect the heart, according to certain research. Polysaccharides found in them have

anti-inflammatory and cholesterol-lowering properties, which may make them less likely to cause cardiovascular disease.

Barley

There are several health advantages to eating barley, a grain that is very nutritious. The following is an exhaustive analysis of its nutritional value and the associated health benefits:

Nutritional Content:

1. **Fiber**: Barley has a lot of fiber, both soluble and insoluble. A decrease in cholesterol and an improvement in blood sugar stability may be achieved with the aid of soluble fiber, namely beta-glucans. By increasing stool size and promoting bowel regularity, insoluble fibers help in digestion.
2. **Minerals and Vitamins:** Energy generation and general health are aided by the B vitamins found in barley, which include niacin, riboflavin, and thiamin. Minerals like as selenium, magnesium, manganese, and phosphorus are essential for a variety of body activities and are also provided by it.
3. **Antioxidants:** Barley contains several phytochemicals and vitamin E, which are known to help shield cells from oxidative stress and may even lower the likelihood of developing chronic illnesses.

Health Benefits:

1. **Supports Heart Health**: The beta-glucan fiber in LDL cholesterol may be reduced by eating barley (the "bad" cholesterol), thereby lowering the risk of heart disease. Antioxidants in barley also contribute to cardiovascular health

by reducing inflammation and preventing damage to blood vessels.

2. **Supports Digestive Health:** Barley's high fiber content encourages regular bowel movements and helps avoid constipation, two symptoms of poor digestion. Additionally, it helps maintain a balanced microbiota in the digestive tract, which is critical to good health in general.
3. **Maintains Healthy Blood Sugar Levels:** The fiber in barley may help regulate blood sugar levels by slowing the absorption of sugar. This makes it a beneficial food for managing diabetes and maintaining stable energy levels.
4. **Weight Management**: If you're trying to control your weight, eating barley may help since its fiber makes you feel full on fewer calories. If your goal is to reduce or maintain your current weight, this will assist.
5. **Supports Bone Health**: The minerals found in barley, such as phosphorus, magnesium, and manganese, contribute to bone health by supporting bone structure and strength

Black pepper

Black pepper, scientifically known as Piper nigrum, is a popular spice that is widely used for its flavor and potential health benefits. The active compound in black pepper, piperine, is responsible for many of its health-promoting properties.

Nutritional Content:

1. **Piperine**: This bioactive compound contains, which gives black pepper its characteristic heat and many health benefits, is an essential ingredient.

2. **Minerals and Vitamins:** Black pepper contains trace levels of iron and a number of minerals, including vitamins C and K potassium.

Health Benefits:

1. **Improves Digestion**: Black pepper promotes better digestion by increasing the production of hydrochloric acid in the stomach. If you're experiencing indigestion or gas, this may assist.
2. it improves nutrient absorption; research has shown that piperine increases the bioavailability of several nutrients. This implies that it may improve the usage and absorption of minerals such as coenzyme Q10, selenium, beta-carotene, and vitamin B6.
3. Anti-inflammatory Properties: Piperine may help lower inflammation in the body due to its anti-inflammatory actions. When dealing with chronic inflammatory disorders, this may help.
4. Black pepper has antioxidant effects: These effects assist the body destroy free radicals. This may lessen the likelihood of developing chronic illnesses by shielding cells from oxidative stress.
5. Possible Positive Effects on Brain Health: Research indicates that piperine has the ability to enhance brain function and provide protection against neurodegenerative disorders via enhancing cognitive function and providing neuroprotective effects

Lion's Mane mashroom:

The medicinal fungus known as Lion's Mane (Hericium erinaceus) has recently gained interest due to claims that it may have positive effects on health, particularly neural regeneration and brain function. A comprehensive analysis of its features and advantages is presented here:

Components:

1. **Hericenones and Erinacines**: This is a list of active ingredients for Lion's Mane mushrooms. Hericenones are typically found in the fruiting body, while erinacines are mainly present in the mycelium. Both compounds are believed to play a crucial role in promoting nerve growth factor (NGF) synthesis.

Health Benefits:

1. **Supports Brain Health**: The reputed cognitive-enhancing properties of Lion's Mane have made it famous. The chemicals hericenones and erinacines have the ability to enhance the synthesis of NGF, a protein that plays a crucial role in the development, upkeep, and survival of neurons, including neurons in the brain. This support can potentially improve memory and cognitive function.
2. **Nerve Regeneration**: The ability of Lion's Mane to boost NGF synthesis suggests it might aid in nerve regeneration. This could be beneficial for individuals with peripheral nerve injury or degenerative neurological diseases.
3. **Potential Anti-Cancer Properties**: According to certain research, Lion's Mane may be able to fight cancer. In vitro studies have shown that mushroom extracts may halt the

proliferation of cancer cells. The antioxidant and immune system-stimulating qualities of this substance may be responsible for these effects.
4. Lion's Mane has powerful antioxidant and anti-inflammatory effects, which brings us to our fourth point. Chronic inflammation and oxidative stress are associated with a host of health problems, including cardiovascular disease and neurological diseases; these characteristics may help shield the body from these threats.
5. Advantages to Mood and Mental Health: Early studies suggest that Lion's Mane might alleviate signs of sadness and anxiety, perhaps via promoting neurogenesis and reducing inflammation

The traditional medicinal herb Piper longum, often called long pepper, contains the bioactive chemical piperine. Because of its medicinal qualities, it has been used in several traditional medical systems for a long time. Here are the key components and health benefits of Piper longum:

Key Components:

1. **Piperine**: This is the most active alkaloid found in Piper longum, responsible for its distinct pungency and several of its health benefits.

Health Benefits:

1. **Aids Digestion**: Piper longum has been traditionally used the digestive process. Piperine boosts the production of digestive enzymes and the bioavailability of nutrients, which facilitates efficient digestion.

2. **Anti-inflammatory Properties**: Piper longum exhibits significant anti-inflammatory properties. It has the potential to alleviate inflammatory diseases by lowering systemic inflammation and promoting overall health.
3. **Analgesic Properties**: The analgesic (pain-relieving) properties of Piper longum make it useful in alleviating numerous forms of discomfort, such as aches and pains in the joints and the brain. Theoretically, it exerts its effects via influencing the body's pain pathways.
4. Piper longum may have antioxidant effects that protect cells from free radical damage, according to some research. As a result, oxidative stress and the likelihood of developing chronic illnesses may be reduced.
5. **Enhanced Nutrient Absorption**: Like black pepper, the piperine in long pepper enhances the absorption of various nutrients and medications, making them more effective

Zingiber officinale:

Zingiber officinale, commonly known as ginger, is a widely used spice and medicinal herb with numerous health benefits. It is particularly known for its effects on digestion, nausea, and inflammation.

Key Components:

1. **Gingerol**: The primary the therapeutic benefits of ginger are attributed to gingerol, a bioactive molecule found in ginger. Significant anti-inflammatory and antioxidant properties are shown by it.

Health Benefits:

1. **Aids Digestion**: Ginger is known to enhance digestive processes. It stimulates the synthesis of digestive enzymes, that may facilitate better food digestion and absorption. In addition to its other uses, it helps with gastrointestinal issues including gas and bloating.
2. **Reduces Nausea**: Ginger is highly effective in reducing nausea and is commonly used to relieve nausea caused by motion sickness, pregnancy (morning sickness), and chemotherapy. Its anti-nausea effects are thought to be due to its ability to influence the digestive and central nervous systems.
3. **Anti-inflammatory Properties**: Conditions like rheumatoid arthritis and osteoarthritis may benefit from ginger's anti-inflammatory properties, which help alleviate inflammation and discomfort. This is attributed to gingerol and other related compounds that inhibit inflammatory pathways in the body.
4. **Antioxidant Effects**: By warding off oxidative stress and damage, ginger's antioxidants promote general health and may even lower the likelihood of developing chronic illnesses.
5. Ginger may have heart-healthy effects, including lowering cholesterol and improving blood sugar management, according to some research.

Green tea

Green tea leaves are renowned for their advantages to health, mainly because of the abundance of catechins, an antioxidant. An in-depth analysis of these advantages may be found here:

catechins, which are antioxidants in nature, help protect cells from harm and have other positive effects on health. Epigallocatechin gallate (EGCG) is the most abundant catechin in green tea and has strong therapeutic effects; it has been the subject of much research.

Increasing one's metabolic rate and decreasing hunger are two ways in which green tea might help one lose weight increasing fat burning, especially during exercise. The catechins, in conjunction with caffeine, enhance thermogenesis, helping the body burn more calories.

1. **Improves Brain Function**: It is possible for green tea's caffeine and L-theanine to improve brain function by enhancing mood, reaction time, and memory. Additionally, catechins may have protective effects on neurons, potentially lowering the risk of neurodegenerative diseases.
2. **Antioxidant Properties**: Green There are a lot of antioxidants in tea, which may help lower oxidative stress by combating free radicals. This can lower the risk of chronic diseases and contribute to overall health and longevity

Asparagus racemosus, commonly known as Shatavari, is an important herb in Ayurvedic medicine, renowned for its ability to support reproductive health and provide antioxidant benefits. The active compounds in Shatavari, such as saponins, are responsible for its therapeutic effects. Take a closer look at these chemicals and the associated health benefits:

1. **Active Compounds - Saponins**: The primary active compounds in Shatavari are steroidal saponins, known as shatavarins. Shatavarin IV is particularly notable for its role in the herb's health benefits. These saponins are believed to

contribute to the adaptogenic, antioxidant, and reproductive health-supporting properties of Shatavari.

2. **Supports Reproductive Health**: Shatavari is traditionally used to support female reproductive health, including regulating menstrual cycles, enhancing fertility, and alleviating symptoms of menopause. It is also used to support lactation in nursing mothers by promoting milk production. These benefits are attributed to Shatavari's ability to balance hormones and its phytoestrogenic propertiess.

3. **Antioxidant Properties**: Shatavari has strong antioxidant properties that aid in free radical neutralization, which in turn protects cells from oxidative stress and harm. As a result, you may live longer and better with fewer chronic conditions. The antioxidants in Shatavari also support immune function, further enhancing its health benefits.

Mentha piperata

Mentha piperata, commonly known as peppermint, is a multipurpose plant that has antibacterial and digestive health effects. A large percentage of peppermint's medicinal value comes from its active ingredients, especially menthol. Examining these substances and the ways in which they contribute to good health:

1. **Active Compound - Menthol**: Menthol is the principal ingredient in peppermint that gives it its cooling effect sensation and aromatic qualities. It is responsible for many of peppermint's medicinal properties, including its effects on the digestive system and its antimicrobial activity

2. **Supports Digestive Health**: Peppermint is widely used to support digestive health. Bloating, gas, and stomach discomfort

are some of the symptoms of irritable bowel syndrome (IBS), which it may help reduce. In instance, research has shown that peppermint oil may ease gastrointestinal spasms and promote more efficient digestion by relaxing the muscles in the digestive system. This makes peppermint a popular natural remedy for indigestion and other digestive discomforts
3. **Antimicrobial Properties**: Peppermint has antimicrobial properties that can help battle against several kinds of germs, viruses, and fungus. Ethanol and other essential oils in peppermint can inhibit the growth of microorganisms, making it useful in treating infections and maintaining oral hygiene. This antimicrobial action contributes to peppermint's use in natural cleaning products and personal care items

Cinnamon

Cinnamon extract is widely recognized for its ability to support blood sugar regulation and provide antioxidant benefits. These health advantages are mostly due to the active chemicals found in cinnamon, particularly cinnamaldehyde. A comprehensive analysis of these chemicals and their effects:

1. **Active Compound - Cinnamaldehyde**: Cinnamaldehyde is the primary active compound in cinnamon, responsible for its distinctive flavor and aroma. It is known for its potential effects on metabolism and its ability to improve insulin sensitivity, which can help regulate blood sugar levels.
2. **Supports Blood Sugar Regulation**: Cinnamon extract has been researched for the beneficial impact it has on glucose levels in the blood. Insulin sensitivity may be improved, decrease insulin resistance, and improve glucose uptake by

cells. These actions contribute to better blood sugar control, particularly beneficial for individuals with type 2 diabetes or at risk for the condition.

Antioxidant Properties: Cinnamon is rich in antioxidants, which help reduce oxidative stress and inflammation in the body. These antioxidants, including polyphenols, can protect cells from damage caused by free radicals, thereby lowering the risk of chronic diseases and supporting overall health.

Boswellia

Boswellia, also known as Indian frankincense, is a herbal extract derived from the Boswellia tree. It is well-regarded for its ability to support joint health and possess anti-inflammatory properties. The key active compounds in Boswellia are boswellic acids, which contribute to its therapeutic effects. Here's a detailed look at these compounds and their health benefits:

1. **Active Compound - Boswellic Acids**: Boswellic acids are the primary active compounds in Boswellia, known for their potent anti-inflammatory effects. Among these, acetyl-11-keto-β-boswellic acid (AKBA) is one of the most studied for its role in inhibiting the enzyme 5-lipoxygenase, which plays a part in the inflammatory process.
2. **Supports Joint Health**: Boswellia is commonly used to support joint health, particularly in conditions like osteoarthritis. It helps reduce joint pain, stiffness, and swelling by decreasing inflammation. This can lead to improved mobility and a better quality of life for individuals with joint issues.

3. **Boswellia's anti-inflammatory activities are believed to be due to** its ability to inhibit pro-inflammatory enzymes and cytokines. This action not only benefits joint health but may also help in managing other inflammatory conditions, such as inflammatory bowel disease and asthma

Ashwagandha:

Active Compounds - Withanolides: The primary active compounds in ashwagandha are withanolides, which are believed to contribute to its adaptogenic and therapeutic effects.

Reduces Stress: Ashwagandha is known for its adaptogenic properties, helping the body manage stress. It can lower cortisol levels, the hormone associated with stress, which may improve stress resilience and reduce anxiety

Enhances Mood: By reducing stress and balancing neurotransmitters, ashwagandha can enhance mood and help alleviate symptoms of depression and anxiety.

Supports Brain Health: Ashwagandha may improve cognitive function and memory by promoting neurogenesis and protecting brain cells from oxidative stress.

Moringa

Active Compounds - Isothiocyanates, Flavonoids: Moringa contains a wide range of bioactive compounds, including isothiocyanates and flavonoids, which contribute to its health benefits.

Rich in Vitamins and Minerals: Moringa is packed with essential nutrients, including vitamins A, C, and E, calcium, potassium, and protein, supporting overall health and nutrition

Supports Overall Health: Due to its nutrient density, moringa supports immune function, energy levels, and overall vitality.

Antioxidant Properties: The antioxidants in moringa, such as quercetin and chlorogenic acid, help reduce oxidative stress and inflammation.

Grape Seed:

Active Compounds - Proanthocyanidins: Grape seed extract is rich in proanthocyanidins, powerful antioxidants that provide a range of health benefits.

Rich in Antioxidants: Proanthocyanidins in grape seed extract are potent antioxidants that help protect cells from oxidative damage and reduce inflammation.

Supports Heart Health: Grape seed extract may improve cardiovascular health by reducing blood pressure, improving blood flow, and lowering cholesterol levels.

Supports Skin Health: Antioxidants in grape seed extract can enhance skin elasticity and reduce signs of aging by protecting against UV damage and promoting collagen synthesis

Passion flower

Passion flower, known botanically as Passiflora incarnata, is valued for its calming effects and various health benefits. The active compounds in passion flower, such as flavonoids and alkaloids, contribute significantly to its therapeutic properties. Here's a detailed look at these compounds and their health benefits:

1. **Active Compounds - Flavonoids and Alkaloids**: Passion flower contains several active compounds, including flavonoids (such as vitexin, apigenin) and alkaloids (such as harmine), which contribute to its calming and health-promoting effects.
2. **Reduces Anxiety**: Passion flower is often used for its sedative effects, which make it an all-natural treatment for nervousness. One theory is that it promotes relaxation by raising brain levels of the neurotransmitter gamma-aminobutyric acid (GABA).
3. **Supports Sleep**: By promoting relaxation and decreasing anxiety, passion flower can help improve sleep quality and is often used to treat insomnia. It allows for a more restful sleep by reducing overactive thoughts and calming the nervous systeme.
4. **Anti-inflammatory and Pain Relief**: Research has shown that passion flower might potentially have anti-inflammatory properties, which can help relieve pain and reduce inflammation associated with conditions like arthritis

Angelica gigas:

Angelica gigas, commonly known as Korean angelica, giant angelica, purple parsnip, and dangquai, is a robust biennial or short-lived perennial plant native to Korea, China, and Japan. It thrives in moist, loamy soil and prefers partial shade. The plant is characterized by its stout stature, reaching up to 1 to 2 meters in height, with deep thick roots and a purplish, ribbed stem. Its large, deeply dissected leaves are broad and pointy.

Angelica gigas is valued for its purple flowers and reddish-purple stems, which are not only attractive but also serve as a food source for bees, butterflies, and birds. The plant is known for its large, domed scented dark red flower-heads that bloom in August. It is also appreciated for its architectural qualities, making it suitable for large borders or naturalizing in woodland settings.

In traditional Chinese medicine, the roots of Angelica gigas are used, and the plant has been studied for its chemical components, including the coumarin derivative decursin, which has been found to have anti-androgenic properties in vitro. Additionally, the plant is used in Korea as a blood tonic and to treat women's complaints.

Key components of Angelica gigas include:

1. **Polysaccharides**: These are complex carbohydrates that have been shown in order to modulate the immune system and maybe strengthen the body's defenses.
2. Phthalides are a class of chemicals with anti-inflammatory and vasodilatory effects; two examples are butylphthalide and sedanolide, potentially aiding in improved blood circulation.
3. **Coumarins**: Compounds such as decursin and decursinol angelate have been identified in Angelica gigas. These substances are being studied for their possible ability to fight cancer particularly in hormone-dependent cancers.
4. **Ferulic acid**: This is an antioxidant that have the ability to shield cells from free radical damage, thereby decreasing the likelihood of developing chronic illnesses.
5. **Lignans**: These are phytoestrogens that may have a role in hormone regulation and undergo research to see if they

alleviate menopausal symptoms and other hormone-related disorders.

Health benefits:

1. **Hormonal Balance**: Due to its phytoestrogen content, Angelica gigas is often used to help balance hormones, particularly in women. It may relieve hot flashes, nocturnal sweats, and other menopausal symptoms.
2. **Blood Circulation**: The vasodilatory properties of Angelica gigas can help improve blood circulation, potentially relieving symptoms of impaired circulation and lowering the risk of cardiovascular diseases, such as cold hands and feet.
3. **Anti-inflammatory Effects**: The phthalides and other compounds in Angelica gigas have been shown helps relieve symptoms of inflammatory disorders and decrease inflammation in the body due to its anti-inflammatory qualities.
4. **Immune Support**: The polysaccharides in Angelica gigas may assist in regulating the immune system, which may improve the body's inherent defenses.
5. Ferulic acid and other antioxidants support antioxidant defenses, which in turn lower the risk of chronic illnesses including cancer and heart disease by preventing oxidative stress.
6. **Digestive Health**: Traditional employing Angelica gigas includes aiding in digestion and relieving gastrointestinal discomfort.

7. **Pain Relief**: Some components of Angelica gigas ongoing research into their analgesic properties suggests they might be useful in pain relief, particularly menstrual pain.

Cinnamomum zeylanicum:

The inner bark of the Cinnamomum zeylanicum tree is the source of cinnamon, which goes by many names: Ceylon cinnamon, "true" cinnamon, and others. This is distinguished from other types of cinnamon, such as cassia, by its more delicate flavor and its health benefits, which are supported by various scientific studies.

Key Components:

Cinnamaldehyde: This is mostly responsible for giving cinnamon its distinctive fragrance and taste. Many of cinnamon's purported health advantages are thought to be attributed to it as well.

Polyphenols: These are powerful antioxidants that contribute to cinnamon's health benefits3.

Antioxidants: The abundance of antioxidants in cinnamon aids in preventing oxidative damage to cells.

Health Benefits:

Anti-inflammatory Properties: Cinnamon is associated with a decreased incidence of chronic illnesses because to its anti-inflammatory actions.

Blood Sugar Control: It can aid diabetics by lowering blood sugar levels and increasing insulin sensitivity 312.

Cardiovascular Health: Cinnamon's ability to reduce cholesterol and blood pressure makes it a potential risk factor for cardiovascular disease.

Cinnamon's antimicrobial effects and antioxidant properties make it a promising natural preservative.

Cinnamon's strong antioxidant levels help protect against oxidative stress and lower the risk of certain illnesses.

Japanese fern:

The Japanese peony, or Paeonia japonica, is a kind of herbaceous peony that originated in Japan to certain islands in northern Japan. It is characterized by its compact size and single flowers, making it a popular choice for woodland gardens.

Key Components

Paeonia japonica, like other peony species, contains various chemical components that give it its therapeutic benefits. These include:

1. **Paeoniflorin**: A chemical found in peony that has undergone research about its possible use in the topical reduction of face wrinkles.
2. **Peelomyrtins**: These substances have anti-inflammatory and immunomodulatory effects5.
3. **Other Compounds**: Including antioxidants and additional phytochemicals that enhance peony's health advantages generally.

Health Benefits

The health benefits of Paeonia japonica, similar to other peony species, include:

1. **Anti-inflammatory and Immunomodulatory Effects**: Peony rheumatoid arthritis and systemic lupus erythematosus are two illnesses that may benefit from its traditional usage of reducing inflammation and modulating the immune system.
2. **Part Two:** Antioxidant Capabilities: The antioxidant chemicals found in peony help shield cells from free radical damage and may even lower the likelihood of developing some debilitating illnesses.
3. **Analgesic and Anti-spasmodic Effects**: Peony is used to alleviate pain and muscle spasms, making it useful for conditions like menstrual cramps and muscle spasms associated with liver cirrhosis.
4. **Hemorrhoids**: Applied topically, peony can help heal cracked skin, particularly around the anus, which is common with hemorrhoids

Panax ginseng:

Traditional medicine in East Asian nations makes extensive use of the highly prized plant panax ginseng, most often known as Korean ginseng. For thousands of years, people have turned to it as a remedy for a wide range of health issues, according to its legendary properties.

Key Components

The triterpene saponins known as ginsenosides are the principal active ingredients in Panax ginseng. These compounds are categorized into three types based on their chemical structure: oleanolic acid type, dammarane type, and oleanane type. Of the several ginsenosides, the ones that have received the most attention from researchers are Rb1, Rb2, Rc, Rd, Re, and Rg1.

Health Benefits

1. **Immune System**: Panax ginseng has been shown to enhance immune function, making it a valuable herb for maintaining a healthy immune system.
2. **Cancer**: It exhibits anti-cancer properties by inhibiting the activation of immune resistance and cancer metastasis via NF-κB, which considerably reduces the expression of MMPs, Snail, Slug, TWIST1, and PD-L1.
3. **Heart and Vascular Wellness:** Cardiovascular illnesses like heart failure, atherosclerosis, and ischemia reperfusion damage are protected against by ginsenosides by improving energy metabolism and inhibiting hyperlipidemia.
4. **Neurodegenerative Diseases**: There is substantial evidence supporting Panax ginseng's potential health benefits in awarding against neurodegeneration.
5. **Antioxidant Effects**: Ginsenosides have antioxidant properties, that lessen the likelihood of developing chronic illnesses by fighting oxidative stress.
6. Panax ginseng is a favorite among athletes since it helps them maintain high energy levels and physical endurance and those engaged in strenuous physical activities.

7. **Diabetes**: It has been studied for its possibility for enhancing insulin sensitivity and decreasing blood glucose levels in the context of diabetes management.
8. **Mental Health**: Ginseng may help in reducing symptoms of anxiety and depression

Milk Thistle:

An annual blooming plant of the Asteraceae family, milk thistle is formally known as Silybum marianum. It has long stems topped with distinctive purple blooms and big, spiky foliage. This plant originally hails from the Mediterranean but is now a global invasive weed due to its rapid proliferation.

Key Components:

The primary active compound in milk thistle is silymarin, a complex of flavonoids including silybin, silydianin, and silychristin. Silymarin is known for its potent antioxidant and anti-inflammatory properties.

Health Benefits:

1. **Liver Health**: Milk thistle is renowned for its ability to protect and regenerate liver cells. Its usage in the treatment of liver disorders dates back centuries such as cirrhosis, jaundice, and hepatitis. Silymarin, the active compound in milk thistle, has been shown to enhance The liver protects itself from harmful substances, fights free radicals, and keeps scars from forming.
2. **Diabetes Management**: Milk thistle may help It is advantageous for those with diabetes or at risk of acquiring

the disease since it regulates insulin levels and maintains balanced blood sugar levels.

3. it promotes heart health due to its high levels of omega-3 fatty acids and other beneficial fatty acids. Atherosclerosis may be prevented with the aid of omega-3 fatty acids by maintaining normal cholesterol levels.
4. **Regulating Cholesterol:** Milk thistle has anti-inflammatory properties and aids in lowering cholesterol levels, which improves cardiovascular health.
5. **Reduced Risk of Gallstones:** Milk thistle prevents gallstones by improving the function of the gallbladder, kidneys, and spleen and by flushing the body of metabolic waste. Sixth, for skin care, milk thistle's anti-inflammatory and antioxidant properties help keep skin looking young and healthy.
6. **Weight reduction:** Milk thistle contains silymarin, which is believed to aid with weight reduction.
7. It enhances bone health, which lowers the risk of osteoporosis, and helps prevent bone loss caused by an estrogen deficit.
8. Milk thistle's silymarin helps alleviate allergic asthma symptoms by lowering airway inflammation.
9. **Improved Immunity:** Milk thistle promotes glutathione synthesis in the body, which increases general immunity and fights against infections, which helps fight oxidative stress.
10. **Anti-fungal Activity**: Milk thistle has been shown to neutralize certain fungal infections, which is traditionally used as a remedy for mushroom poisoning.
11. **Psoriasis Treatment**: Milk thistle's silymarin content makes it an effective psoriasis therapy.

Crataeva nurvala:

Crataeva nurvala, this plant, which is sometimes called Varuna, is really a member of the Capparidaceae family. Traditional medical systems like Ayurveda, Unani, and Siddha make extensive use of it for its various health benefits.

Key Components:

Alkaloids, Triterpenes, Tannins, Saponins, Flavonoids, Plant Sterols, Glucosinolates

Health Benefits:

- **Diuretic:** Helps in increasing urine production, which is useful while dealing with kidney stones and infections of the urinary system.
- **Antilithiatic:** Aids in preventing the formation of urinary stones.
- **Rubefacient:** Has a warming effect on the skin, which can be beneficial for certain skin condition.
- **Anti-inflammatory:** Helps in reducing inflammation in the body.
- **Anti-diabetic:** May help in managing blood sugar levels.
- **Anti-nociceptive:** Has pain-relieving properties.
- **Anti-diarrheal:** Useful in treating diarrhea.
- **Anti-fertility:** May have contraceptive effects.
- **Anti-pyretic:** Helps in reducing fever.
- **Anti-cancer:** Shows potential in preventing cancer.
- **Protection against Oxidative Stress:** Restores antioxidant enzymes and modulates gene expression associated with oxidative stress.

- Urinary Tract Health: Improves urinary tract health and relieves urinary symptoms of BPH (Benign Prostatic Hyperplasia).
- Antimicrobial: Possesses antimicrobial properties.
- Antioxidant: Contains antioxidants that help in fighting free radicals.
- Contraceptive: May have contraceptive effects.
- Anti-periodic: Useful in treating periodic diseases.
- Waste Elimination: Assists in the process of garbage removal.
- Breathing and Lung Problems: May help in respiratory and lung issues.
- Fever: Helps in reducing fever.
- Metabolic Disorders: May be beneficial in metabolic disorders.
- Weak Immunity: Helps in boosting the immune system.
- Joint Lubrication: May help in joint lubrication.
- Skin Problems: Useful in treating skin issues.

Flaxseed:

Flaxseed, also known as linseed, is the tiny seed of the Linum usitatissimum plant, which may be brown or golden in color. It has a long history of medicinal usage due to its high nutritional content and widespread cultural acceptance.

Key Components:

1. **Omega-3 Fatty Acids**: Omega-3 fatty acids are important for human health, and flaxseed has a lot of them, especially alpha-linolenic acid (ALA) cannot be produced by the body.

2. **Lignans**: These are plant compounds with antioxidant properties, which are particularly high in flaxseed.
3. **Fiber**: Flaxseed contains dietary fiber, both soluble and insoluble, that supports a healthy digestive system.
4. It is rich in plant-based protein and a great source of protein overall.
5. Flaxseed is an excellent source of several vitamins and minerals, including folate, selenium, copper, manganese, magnesium, phosphorus, and thiamine.

Health Benefits:
1. **Heart Health**: Flaxseed can help reduce the danger of cardiovascular disease, raise good cholesterol levels, and normalize blood pressure by raising good cholesterol and reducing inflammation.
2. **Digestive Health**: You may say goodbye to constipation and hello to better bowel motions because to flaxseed's high fiber content support overall digestive health.
3. **Cancer Prevention**: Flaxseed's lignans for their possible ability to lower the risk of several malignancies, especially breast cancer, have been researched, by slowing the growth of tumors.
4. **Blood Sugar Control**: Flaxseed can help improve improve insulin sensitivity and lower blood sugar levels, both of which are helpful in diabetes management.
5. **Optimal Skin Health:** Flaxseed's omega-3 fatty acids are known to alleviate skin irritation and promote overall skin health.
6. **Weight control:** Flaxseed's high fiber content aids weight control by making you feel full on fewer calories.

Shilajit:

Shilajit is a natural substance derived from the Himalayan and Tibetan Mountain ranges, where it is formed from the slow decomposition of plants over centuries. Its vast variety of health advantages and distinctive composition have made it famous.

Essential Elements of Shilajit:

1. **Fulvic Acid**: This is the primary active component of shilajit, well-known for the anti-inflammatory and antioxidant effects it has. The use of fulvic acid is beneficial because in preventing the accumulation of tau proteins, which can lead to brain cell damage and is associated with conditions like Alzheimer's disease.
2. **Humic Acid**: Another significant component, humic acid, contributes to the shilajit health advantages, which include improved nutrient absorption and general health support.
3. **Minerals**: Shilajit is beneficial for health since it contains a variety of minerals, including calcium, iron, selenium, and zinc.

Health Benefits of Shilajit:

- **Energy Boost**: Shilajit is known to enhance energy levels enhance energy and stamina, and lessen weariness, making it a well-liked vitamin.
- **Cognitive Health**: The fulvic acid in shilajit supports cognitive health by halting the buildup of tau proteins that cause dementia and other brain cell injuries.

- shilajit may aid in reducing inflammation because of its anti-inflammatory characteristics managing conditions like asthma, allergies, eczema, and diabetes.
- **Bone Health**: It may be beneficial for bone health, potentially aiding in conditions like osteoporosis.
- **Anticancer Properties**: There is some evidence that shilajit may inhibit the growth of certain cancer cells, although more research is needed.
- **Digestive Health**: Fulvic acid in shilajit can improve gut health by increasing good bacteria and enhancing digestive enzyme activity.
- **Stress and Anxiety**: Shilajit has shown in animal experiments the ability to alleviate stress and anxiety, suggesting potential benefits for humans.
- **Antioxidant Properties**: The high concentration of antioxidants in shilajit can help in fighting free radicals and support healthy aging.
- **Heart Health**: Shilajit can improve good cardiovascular health via regulating blood pressure and increasing blood flow.
- **Sexual Health**: It's said to boost testosterone levels in males and improve sexual performance.

19

BALANCING MINERAL INTAKE

The human body relies on minerals, which are inorganic elements, for a wide range of physiological processes. Having strong bones, teeth, and tissues depends on them, as well as for regulating body processes such as metabolism and nerve function. Here's a detailed look at some key minerals:

Calcium:

Function: Bone health depends on calcium, the body's most prevalent mineral. Additionally, it is involved in the process of blood clotting, neuron activity, and muscular contraction.

Calcium Absorption: Vitamin D improves the absorption of calcium. Vitamin D must be present in sufficient amounts for the body to absorb calcium effectively.

Deficiency: Conditions like osteoporosis in adults and rickets in youngsters may result from a lack of calcium.

How Much to Take: The RDA for calcium changes depending on the gender and age group. For instance, whereas the recommended daily allowance (RDA) for adults is usually approximately 1000 mg, it rises to 1200-1400 mg for women who have gone through menopause.

Original Materials: Milk, cheese, and yoghurt are some of the best dairy products for getting the calcium your body needs. Fortified meals, calcium-set tofu, and leafy green vegetables are a few other sources.

Phosphorus:

Function: Phosphorus is a component of bones and teeth, and the creation of energy and the synthesis of crucial molecules, like as DNA, are also facilitated by it and RNA.

Absorption: Phosphorus absorption is aided by vitamin D and calcium.

Deficiency: Phosphorus very seldom, but when it does occur, it may cause teeth and bones to become weak, as well as issues with energy metabolism.

Sources: Phosphorus is widely available in foods such as dairy products, meat, fish, eggs, grains, and legumes.

Iron:

Function: Iron is essential for the production of hemoglobin, a protein found in red blood cells that transports oxygen throughout the body.

Vitamin C improves iron absorption, but phytates, which are included in whole grains and legumes, decrease it.

A lack of iron in the body may cause anemia, which manifests as a lack of energy, weakness, and a pale complexion.

Recommended Dosage: The RDA for iron varies significantly with age, gender, and physiological state (e.g., pregnancy). For example, daily dosage for males is around 8 mg, while for women before menopause it's 18 mg.

Original Materials: The following foods are rich in iron: red meat, chicken, fish, lentils, beans, tofu, iron-fortified cereals, and dark greens.

Magnesium:

Function: Muscle and neuron function, blood glucose management, and blood pressure regulation are just a few of the more than 300 metabolic events in which magnesium participates in the body.

Absorption: Magnesium absorption is influenced by dietary fiber, which can bind to magnesium and decrease its absorption.

Deficiency: Muscle cramps, lethargy, arrhythmia, and mood swings are all symptoms of magnesium shortage.

Dosage Recommendation: Men should take 400–420 mg of magnesium daily, while women should take 310–320 mg.

The following foods are good sources of magnesium: nuts (particularly cashews and almonds), seeds (including sunflower and pumpkin seeds), whole grains, legumes, and dark greens.

Thyroid hormones control metabolism, growth, and development; iodine is necessary for their creation. Inadequate iodine intake may cause hypothyroidism, goiter, and developmental problems in kids.

Eggs, shellfish, and dairy products are good sources of iodine. A substantial amount of iodine may also be found in iodized salt.

Red blood cells and connective tissue cannot be formed without copper. Copper also aids in energy synthesis and iron absorption.

Absorption: Copper absorption is influenced by the amount of copper in the diet, as well as by other dietary components like zinc and vitamin C.

Deficiency: Copper anemia and neurological issues are some outcomes of a deficit.

Where to Find It: Shellfish, nuts, seeds, and whole grains are just a few of the many dietary sources of copper.

Zinc:

Function: Zinc is involved in the process of carbohydrate breakdown, wound healing, cell proliferation, and cell division. It is involved in immune system function as well.

Absorption: Zinc absorption is influenced by dietary phytates and can be inhibited by high intakes of calcium and iron.

Deficiency: Zinc deficiency can lead to growth retardation, skin changes, and impaired immune function.

Recommended Dosage: Adult males should consume 11 milligrams of zinc per day and 8 mg per adult female.

Original Materials: Some of the many foods that contain zinc include lean meats, seafood, nuts, seeds, and whole grains.

While these minerals are necessary for good health, it's worth noting that too much of them might be dangerous. For example, too much calcium can lead to kidney stones, while excessive iron can cause liver damage. Thus, it is essential to get the required minerals in your diet and to seek the counsel of a healthcare professional or a certified dietitian for specific dietary recommendations.

Vitamins are natural substances that the body needs in tiny amounts for proper development and nourishment but cannot produce on its own. Vitamins play an essential role in the body by facilitating metabolic activities. They help the immune system function properly, keep the skin and eyes healthy, control cell development and division, and make sure that food is turned into energy efficiently.

The human body requires thirteen different vitamins, four of which are fat-soluble (vitamins A, D, E, and K) and six of which are water-soluble (vitamin C and the B-complex vitamins B1, B2, B3, B5, B6, B7, B9, and B12).

Here's a detailed look at each vitamin, considering their function, absorption, deficiency, recommended dosage, and sources:

Fat-Soluble Vitamins

Vitamin A

Function: Essential in order to facilitate cellular communication, eyesight, immunological function, and reproduction.

Bile salts and dietary lipids aid absorption in the small intestine.

Insufficiency: Problems seeing at night, skin that is dry, and an increased risk of infection.

Recommended Dosage: For adults, the recommended dietary allowance (RDA) amounts to 700 mcg for females and 900 mcg for males.

Sources: Liver, fish oil, sweet potatoes, carrots, spinach, kale, and broccoli.

Vitamin D

Function: The mineral phosphorus and the mineral calcium are both essential for strong bones, and this aids in their absorption.

Bile salts and dietary lipids aid absorption in the small intestine.

Inadequate levels: rickets in kids, osteomalacia in grownups, brittle bones, and compromised immune system.

Recommended Dosage: The RDA for adults is 600 International Units (IU) for those under 70 years and 800 IU for those over 70.

Sources: The sun, fatty fish, fortified dairy products, egg yolks, mushrooms, and other similar resources.

Vitamin E is essential for immune system functioning and functions as an antioxidant, preventing cell damage.

Absorption: Absorbed to the small intestine with the assistance of bile salts and dietary fats.

Deficiency: Rare but can lead to hemolytic anemia and neurological issues.

Recommended Dosage: The RDA Day for adults is fifteen milligrams (mg).

Here are several sources: avocados, nuts, seeds, spinach, and vegetable oils.

Blood coagulation and bone metabolism are two of vitamin K's essential functions.

Bile salts and dietary lipids aid absorption in the small intestine.

Bleeding problems, excessive menstrual bleeding, and easy bruising are symptoms of a deficiency.

How Much to Take: The recommended daily allowance (RDA) for adults is 90 mcg for women and 120 mcg for men.

Sources: Green leafy vegetables, broccoli, Brussels sprouts, and soybeans.

Water-Soluble Vitamins

Vitamin C

Function: Serves as an antioxidant, helps the immune system work, and is essential for making

of collagen.

Absorption: Absorbed in the small intestine; absorption can be enhanced by consuming smaller doses throughout the day.

Deficiency: Scurvy, characterized by bleeding gums, joint pain, and skin lesions.

Recommended Dosage: Adults should not exceed 90 mg for males and 75 mg for women.

Fruits and vegetables such as strawberries, kiwis, bell peppers, broccoli, and Brussels sprouts are the sources.

B-Complex Vitamins

Vitamin B1 (Thiamine)

Function: Essential for energy metabolism and nerve function.

Absorption: Transmitted to the small intestine.

Deficiency: Beriberi, characterized by muscle weakness and nerve damage.

Recommended Dosage: As an adult, a man should take 1.2 mg and a woman 1.1 mg.

Ingredients: Pork, nuts, seeds, lentils, and whole grains. A vitamin called riboflavin

Purpose: Crucial for the generation of energy, maintenance of eyesight, and antioxidant defense. The small intestine is responsible for absorption.

Deficiency: Ariboflavinosis, characterized by sore throat, redness of the mouth, and skin issues.

Recommended Dosage: As an adult, a man should consume 1.3 mg and a woman 1.1 mg.

Ingredients: Eggs, dairy, lean meats, and leafy greens.

Vitamin B3 (Niacin)

Function: Crucial for proper nerve and energy system function, DNA synthesis, and energy metabolism.

The small intestine is the site of absorption.

Deficiency: Pellagra, characterized by diarrhea, dermatitis, and dementia.

Recommended Dosage: The RDA for adults is (16 mg for males and 14 mg for females).

Ingredients: Legumes, nuts, meat, chicken, fish, and whole grains.

Anti-Oxidantonism, B5 Vitamin

Role: Crucial in regulating metabolic energy levels and producing essential lipids, cholesterol, and steroid hormones.

Absorption: Small intestine absorption.

Shortcoming: Infrequent but can lead to fatigue, numbness, and tingling.

Recommended Dosage: The RDA for adults is 5 mg.

Sources: Meat, whole grains, avocados, and dairy products.

Vitamin B6 (Pyridoxine)

Function: Essential for amino acid metabolism, red blood cell production, and brain development.

Absorption: Absorbed in the small intestine.

Deficiency: Anemia, skin problems, and neurological issues.

Recommended Dosage: Men should take 1.3 mg per day, while women should take 1.5 mg.

Sources: Poultry, fish, potatoes, chickpeas, and bananas.

Vitamin B7 (Biotin)

Function: Important for fatty acid synthesis, glucose metabolism, as well as the condition of one's hair and skin.

Absorption: Absorbed in the small intestine.

Deficiency: Rare but can lead to skin rash, hair loss, and neurological symptoms.

Recommended Dosage: The RDA for adults is 30 mcg.

Sources: Eggs, nuts, seeds, and whole grains.

The function of vitamin B9, also known as folate or folic acid, is to prevent neural tube abnormalities in fetuses, aid in cell division, and synthesis of DNA.

Absorption: Absorbed in the small intestine.

Deficiency: Megaloblastic anemia, neural tube defects in fetuses, at a higher risk for cardiovascular disease.

Recommended Dosage: The RDA for adults is 400 micrograms (mcg).

Sources: Leafy green vegetables, legumes, nuts, and fortified grains.

Vitamin B12 (Cobalamin)

Function: Crucial for the production of DNA, RBCs, and the upkeep of the myelin sheath.

Absorption: Helped absorption in the small intestine by the protein intrinsic factor produced by the stomach.

Deficiency: Pernicious anemia, neurological damage, and fatigue.

Recommended Dosage: Adults should not exceed 2.4 mcg.

Originating from: Protein-rich meats, seafood, dairy, and fortified grains.

Note that vitamins are essential for health, but that a balanced diet, not pills, is the best way to get them. Since the body stores fat-soluble vitamins (A, D, E, and K) in excess, taking in too much of these might be harmful. The excretion of water-soluble vitamins (such as the B-complex and C vitamins) makes them less harmful.

20

THE MULTIDIMENSIONAL BENEFITS OF NATURAL HONEY AND ITS DERIVATIVES

*N*atural honey is a remarkable substance produced by bees through a complex process that begins with the collection of nectar from flowers or secretions from living parts of plants. This nectar is then transformed into honey through a series of steps that include regurgitation, enzymatic breakdown, and evaporation. The bees store the resulting thick, sweet liquid in honeycombs, where it continues to ripen and is eventually harvested by beekeepers.

Composition and Nutritional Value

Honey is composed primarily of carbohydrates, mainly in the form of glucose and fructose, with other components such as water, minerals, vitamins, enzymes, and antioxidants. Depending on the flowers used and the area in which the honey is made, the exact ingredients might differ greatly. One example is the well-known high concentration of methylglyoxal (MGO) in New Zealand's manuka honey which is responsible for its potent antibacterial properties.

Health Benefits

Antioxidant Properties

Honey contains several antioxidants, which assist the body deal with free radical oxidative stress. Cell damage and the onset of chronic illnesses including cancer, heart disease, and neurological problems are both facilitated by these free radicals. Honey contains enzymes, phenolic acids, and flavonoids, all of which act as antioxidants like catalase and peroxidase.

Wound Healing

Healing wounds with honey is an old practice that has been practiced by many cultures. Because of the components it contains, including hydrogen peroxide, it has antimicrobial capabilities like MGO, help prevent infection. Additionally, honey has a high viscosity and low pH, creating an environment that is unfavorable for bacterial growth. It also promotes the formation of granulation tissue, which is essential for wound repair.

Cough Suppression

Honey may help alleviate cough symptoms, according to many studies, especially in kids. For nighttime cough relief, honey works better than over-the-counter cough medicine, according to research published in the Archives of Pediatrics & Adolescent Medicine improving sleep quality in children.

Antibacterial and Antifungal Properties

Honey's low moisture content and acidic pH, along with its production of hydrogen peroxide, create a hostile environment for bacteria and fungi. Certain types of honey, like manuka honey, have is effective against a broad variety of infections, even those that have developed resistance to antibiotics, because to its very potent antibacterial characteristics.

Sensitive Insulin Level

Because of its lower glycemic index (GI), honey has less of an effect on blood sugar levels than refined sugar. Because of this, it is a better option for diabetics, however they should still limit its consumption because of the high sugar level.

Benefits and Implementations

Honey is not only used as a sweetener in a variety of culinary applications but also finds use in traditional and modern medicine. It is used in wound dressings, cough syrups, and in place of artificial sweeteners in cooking and drinking. Because of its antimicrobial and hydrating characteristics, honey is often used in skin care products.

Honey, in its natural form, is a multipurpose sweetener that also happens to be nutrition dense and beneficial to your health in many other ways.

Its antioxidant properties, wound-healing capabilities, cough-suppressing effects, and antibacterial and antifungal properties make Including it in your diet is a smart move. Honey has many health advantages, but to get the most out of it, it's best to ingest moderate amounts of high-quality, pure honey.

Bee pollen

Bee pollen is a nutrient-rich substance that bees collect from flowering plants. It is a crucial source of nutrients for the hive, containing a wide array of vitamins, minerals, proteins, amino acids, and enzymes. This diverse composition makes bee pollen one of nature's most complete foods, offering numerous health benefits to humans.

Composition and Nutritional Value

Bee pollen is formed when bees collect pollen grains from the stamens of flowers. They mix this pollen with nectar and enzymes from their bodies, forming small pellets that are attached to the bees' hind legs and carried back to the hive. These pellets are then used as a nutritional source for the hive, especially during times when nectar is scarce.

The nutritional profile of bee pollen is impressive. It is rich in:

- **Proteins**: Bee pollen contains about 20-35% protein, this is a great way to get the amino acids that your body needs to make proteins.
- It has every one of the necessary amino acids, which the human body needs but cannot create, therefore eating it is the only way to get them.

- Vitamins: Folic acid, vitamin E, bee pollen, and the B-complex vitamins are all found in abundance in bee pollen.
- Minerals: It's a good source of several different minerals, such as selenium, magnesium, calcium, and potassium.
- Enzymes aid in nutrition digestion and absorption.
- Antioxidants: Bee pollen is rich in carotenoids and flavonoids, two types of antioxidants that help keep the body safe from free radical damage.

Health Benefits

Boosting Energy Levels

Bee pollen is often touted as a natural energy booster. Its combination of carbohydrates, proteins, and B-vitamins provides a sustained release of energy; thus, it is a great supplement for anyone wishing to enhance their endurance and stamina.

Improving Athletic Performance

The high nutritional content of bee pollen, including its protein and amino acid profile, may aid in the regeneration and development of muscles, leading to better performance in sports. It may also help reduce inflammation and muscle soreness post-exercise.

Supporting Heart Health

The antioxidants in bee pollen can help reduce variables that increase the likelihood of cardiovascular disease, including oxidative stress and inflammation. Having heart-healthy minerals like folic acid and potassium on hand also helps bring blood pressure down and lowers the risk of cardiovascular illnesses.

Other Potential Benefits

Bee pollen has also been credited along with a host of other health advantages, such as:

Helps the Immune System: Bee pollen is rich in minerals and vitamins, which the body uses to fight off illness.

For those who suffer from allergies, there is some evidence that eating local bee pollen might alleviate symptoms by building a tolerance to the allergens over time.

Bee pollen's antioxidants are great for your skin since they keep it healthy and delay the aging process.

Weight control: Bee pollen's high protein and fiber content may aid weight control by making you feel full for longer and reducing appetite.

Considerations

While bee pollen offers numerous health benefits, its effectiveness can vary depending on several factors:

Individual Variation: People may respond differently to bee pollen based on their individual health status, diet, and lifestyle.

Quality of Pollen: The health benefits of bee pollen can vary depending on its quality, which is affected by things like where the pollen came from, how it is collected, and how it is stored.

Allergies: Individuals with pollen allergies should exercise caution when consuming bee pollen, as it can cause allergic reactions in sensitive individuals.

Vegetable gel

The royal jelly that bees make is an unusual and very healthy product to feed queen bees and their larvae. This milky secretion is crucial for the development and health of the queen bee, endowing her with increased size, longevity, and reproductive capabilities compared to worker bees. Royal jelly has a wealth of nutrients that have sparked attention about its possible health advantages for humans. These nutrients include amino acids, B-vitamins, and vitamin C.

Ingredients and Health Benefits

Royal jelly is composed of water, proteins, sugars minerals, lipids, and a host of vitamins. Its protein content includes a range of amino acids, both essential and non-essential, which are vital for various bodily functions. The B-vitamins present in royal jelly, such as Essential for cellular health, energy generation, and metabolism are the B vitamins: thiamine (B1), riboflavin (B2), pyridoxine (B6), cobalamin (B12), biotin, and pantothenic acid. Royal jelly also has vitamin C, which aids the immune system and has antioxidant effects.

Health Benefits
Boosting the Immune System

Royal jelly is thought to have immunomodulatory actions, which imply it may aid in immune system regulation and enhancement. The antioxidants in it prevent oxidative stress, which lowers the immune system's defenses. Royal jelly also has chemicals that may make immune cells work better, which means the body is better able to fight off illnesses and infections.

Improving Cognitive Function

A small body of research suggests that royal jelly could improve brain function. The neurotransmitter acetylcholine, which is essential for learning and memory, is present in it. Royal jelly may have neuroprotective properties that help with diseases like Alzheimer's, according to some research. It also improves cognitive ability.

Minimizing Redness

Although the body's inflammatory response is normal in reaction to infections or injuries, long-term inflammation has been linked to the onset of many illnesses, including as cancer, diabetes, and cardiovascular disease. One anti-inflammatory component found in royal jelly is 10-hydroxy-2-decenoic acid (10-HDA). By reducing inflammation, royal jelly may help protect against these chronic conditions.

Other Potential Benefits

Royal jelly has been linked to several other health advantages, such as:

➢ **Antioxidant Properties:** Its anti-aging properties may be due to its ability to shield the skin from free radical damage.

Because of its antimicrobial and anti-inflammatory characteristics, royal jelly may speed up the healing process of wounds ability to stimulate cell growth.

➢ **Hormonal Balance**: Menopausal symptoms and polycystic ovarian syndrome (PCOS) are among the illnesses that royal jelly may alleviate, according to some research.

➤ **Fatigue and Stress Reduction:** Royal jelly is often touted as an energy booster and may help reduce feelings of fatigue and stress.

Scientific Research and Considerations

While royal jelly is believed to offer numerous health benefits, scientific research in this area is limited and further research is required to completely comprehend its impacts. It is challenging to draw firm conclusions from the current research because of the limited sample sizes and methodological variations. Furthermore, variables including product quality, dose, and individual health problems might affect how well royal jelly works.

Royal jelly is a nutrient-rich substance with the potential to offer a variety is associated with a number of positive health effects, including as enhanced immunity, enhanced cognitive function, and decreased inflammation. Nevertheless, further studies are required to establish the best doses for various medical issues and to completely comprehend its impacts. Always check with your doctor before beginning a new supplement regimen and be sure to choose high-quality goods to consume royal jelly, especially for individuals with allergies or existing health conditions.

21

OPTIMIZING YOUR FITNESS ROUTINE

*A*ny movement that improves or maintains a person's level of physical fitness and general health is considered physical exercise. Improving one's cardiovascular health, strength, flexibility, and mental well-being are all benefits of this vital component of a healthy lifestyle.

Important daily exercises for a healthy life include:

Walking is a simple yet effective kind of exercise that is easily accessible to individuals of all ages and fitness levels. Compared to high-impact sports like sprinting or leaping, it is easier on the body's joints, why it is called a low-impact exercise. So, if you want to be in better shape without taking any chances, walking is a great option injury that might come with more intense workouts.

To incorporate the following suggestions into your regular walking regimen:

1. **Set a Goal**: Strive to walk quickly for 30 minutes daily. When you move quickly, you walking at a pace that increases your heart rate and makes you breathe harder than usual, but you should still be able to carry on a conversation.
2. **Break It Up**: If 30 minutes at once seems daunting, break it into shorter segments. Three 10-minute walks or two 15-minute walks can be just as beneficial.
3. **Make It a Habit**: Choose a time of day find what works for you and do your best to maintain it. Regardless of first thing in the morning, during lunch breaks, or after dinner, consistency is key.
4. **Use a Pedometer or Fitness Tracker**: Using these aids, you may monitor your progress and distance, providing motivation and a sense of achievement.
5. **Vary Your Routine**: To keep things new and to work out various muscle groups, try walking in a different path every time.
6. **Invite a Friend**: Walking Participating in an activity with a loved one or friend may enhance the experience and help you stay accountable.
7. **Dress Appropriately**: Wear comfortable clothing and supportive shoes to prevent blisters and joint pain.
8. **Stay Safe**: Be aware of your surroundings, especially if you're walking alone or in an unfamiliar area. Use reflective gear if you jog first thing in the morning or last thing at night.

9. **Pay Attention to Your Body**: If you feel any kind of pain or discomfort, it's important to take a break and, if required, seek the advice of a healthcare practitioner.
10. **Combine with Other Activities**: Incorporate walking with several kinds of physical activity to provide a balanced fitness program. For example, you could walk to the gym and then do a strength training session.

There are several health advantages to include walking in your daily routine, including improved cardiovascular health, better weight management, increased muscle strength and endurance, improved mood, and decreased vulnerability to long-term health problems including diabetes and cardiovascular disease.

Strength Training

Exercising your muscles to contract them against an external force is the foundation of strength training, sometimes called resistance training. You only need to use your body weight to do this, free weights, resistance bands, equipment that use weights. Strength training mainly aims to increase muscular mass, bone density, and general physical strength.

Key Exercises:

Push-ups: Target the chest, shoulders, and triceps. Start with a modified version on your knees if necessary.

Squats: Work the quadriceps, hamstrings, glutes, and core. Use a chair for support if needed.

Lunges: Strengthen the legs and improve balance. Can be done forward, backward, or sideways.

Frequency:

Aim must do weight training at least twice every week.

Give your muscles a day off in between workouts so they may heal.

Tips:

Focus on proper form to prevent injuries.

Gradually increase the difficulty by adding more repetitions or using heavier weights.

Incorporate routines that strengthen the whole body, from the legs and back to the chest, shoulders, arms, and core.

Stretching

Stretching is a must-have for every exercise program. To increase mobility and flexibility, it entails flexing and stretching muscles, ligaments, and tendons. Improving posture and lowering injury risk are two additional benefits of regular stretching.

Extending Techniques:

Static stretching entails maintaining a posture for at least thirty seconds.

Dynamic Stretching: Moving through a range of motion without holding the stretch.

Yoga: A form of exercise that combines stretching with strength and balance poses.

Incorporation:

Stretch daily, either as part of your warm-up before exercise or as a cool-down afterward.

Hold static stretches for at least 30 seconds to allow muscles to relax and lengthen.

Perform dynamic stretches before workouts to prepare your body for movement.

Benefits:

Improves flexibility and reduces muscle tightness.

Enhances performance in physical activities.

Can alleviate muscle soreness and improve recovery.

Cardiovascular Exercise

Exercising in a way that raises your heart rate and respiration rate for an extended length of time is called cardiovascular exercise or aerobic exercise. It is crucial for improving heart health, increasing stamina, and aiding in weight management.

Key Activities:

Running: A high-impact activity that can be done outdoors or on a treadmill.

Cycling: Low-impact and can be done on a stationary bike or outdoors.

Swimming: A low-impact full-body exercise routine.

How long does it last?

Maintain a weekly aerobic exercise level of at least 150 minutes at a moderate intensity.

You may do this by exercising for 30 minutes, five days a week.

Another option is to exercise vigorously for 75 minutes per week.

If you're new to exercising, it's best to start out cautiously and build up to more intense and longer sessions.

Choose activities that you enjoy to maintain motivation.

Monitor your heart rate to ensure you work within a safe and effective zone.

You may build a comprehensive fitness regimen that improves your health and wellness by include these workouts in your daily schedule.

Instructions to be Followed While Exercising

Exercising regularly is essential to good health, but only if you know what you're doing and take the necessary safety measures. The following are the specific steps to ensure a safe and effective workout:

1. Warm-Up

Purpose: A warm-up gradually increases your heart rate and prepares your muscles for activity, reducing the risk of injury.

Duration: Spend 5-10 minutes doing running, cycling, or mild aerobic workouts.

Pay close attention: Incorporate dynamic stretches that reflect the motions you'll be performing during your workout to enhance flexibility and mobility.

2. Hydration

Importance: For peak performance and speedy recovery, staying hydrated is key.

Get plenty of water before working out at least 2 hours before exercising to ensure proper hydration.

During Exercise: Sip water regularly, especially during prolonged or intense workouts.

After Exercise: Rehydrate by drinking water or a sports drink if you've been exercising for over an hour.

3. Proper Attire

Clothing: Put on loose-fitting, airy garments that won't restrict your mobility.

Footwear: Choose appropriate shoes that provide support and cushioning for your chosen activity (e.g., running shoes for jogging, cross-trainers for gym workouts).

Accessories: Consider using gloves for weightlifting, a hat for sun protection, or reflective gear for outdoor activities in low light.

4. Listen to Your Body

Pain vs. Discomfort: The experience of feeling some discomfort as you push your limits, but pay attention to sharp or persistent pain.

Adjust Accordingly: If you experience pain, shortness of breath, dizziness, or nausea, stop exercising and seek medical advice if necessary.

Rest: Allow your body to recover by incorporating rest days into your routine.

5. Cool Down

Purpose: A cool-down helps your body transition from exercise to rest, aiding in recovery and preventing muscle soreness.

Duration: Spend 5-10 minutes doing light aerobic exercises to gradually lower your heart rate.

Stretching: Perform static stretches to help muscles relax and improve flexibility. Hold each stretch for at least 30 seconds.

6. Consistency

Regularity: Aim for regular exercise to achieve and maintain fitness goals.

Rest Days: Allow for at least one or two rest days per week to prevent overtraining and promote recovery.

Variety: To avoid monotony and target different muscle areas, mix up your workout routine.

7. Consult a Professional

New to Exercise: If you have never exercised before or haven't done it in a while, consult a fitness professional to design a suitable program.

Health Concerns: Before beginning an exercise program, see your doctor if you have any preexisting diseases or problems.

Personalized Plan: A professional can help tailor an exercise cater to your unique requirements while guaranteeing its efficacy and safety.

22

SPECTRUM OF ALTERNATIVE THERAPIES

Alternative therapies, also known as complementary or integrative medicine, encompass a variety of practices that are not addressed by mainstream medicine. These treatments may be administered alone or in addition to more conventional medical procedures. It should be mentioned that the effectiveness of different treatments might vary, and some might not have strong scientific backing. Listed below are a few other treatment options:

An integral part of TCM, which has been around for more than 2000 years, is acupuncture. It is deeply rooted in the ancient Chinese philosophy that health and wellness are achieved through the balanced flow of Qi (chi), a vital life force or energy that is believed to circulate through the body. According to TCM, Qi flows through specific pathways known as meridians, and disruptions any obstructions in this pathway may cause discomfort, inefficiency, and disease.

Origin

The first documented accounts of acupuncture date to the Han Dynasty (206 BC - 220 AD), establishing its roots in ancient China. The Huangdi Neijing, also known as the Yellow Emperor's Classic of Internal Medicine, provides a comprehensive overview of traditional Chinese medicine (TCM) and its guiding principles, including acupuncture sites, meridians, and Qi.

Theory

Maintaining a steady flow of Qi is the theoretical underpinning of acupuncture. TCM practitioners believe that there are 12 main meridians and numerous branching channels that transport Qi and blood throughout the body, connecting internal organs and the surface of the body. Each meridian is associated with a specific organ and a particular aspect of the body's functions.

When Qi is flowing freely and harmoniously, the body is in a state of health. Nevertheless, signs of emotional, mental, or bodily Qi blockage or imbalance might be discernible. Restoring this equilibrium is the goal of acupuncture, which involves stimulating certain sites along the meridians.

Practice

The practice of acupuncture involves inserting tiny, sterilized needles into specific anatomical sites called acupoints. These specific locations are along the meridians and are believed to be areas where Qi can be accessed and influenced. The insertion of needles is thought to promote the free flow of Qi, correct imbalances, and restore health.

The technique of needle insertion is precise and requires specialized training. Practitioners may manipulate the needles manually or use electrical stimulation to enhance their effects. Sessions typically last from 20 to 40 minutes, as well as the individual's reaction to treatment, the quantity of treatments needed to alleviate a certain disease might differ.

Applications

Acupuncture is used in order to address several medical issues. The following are examples of widespread usage:

Back pain, neck pain, and arthritis are among the many chronic pains that acupuncture may help ease.

Reducing nausea and vomiting is one of its primary uses, especially for chemotherapy patients.

- **Nerve Pain**: Conditions such as sciatica and neuropathy can be addressed with acupuncture.
- **Mental Health**: Acupuncture is effective in alleviating symptoms of sleeplessness, despair, and anxiety.
- **Digestive Issues**: It can help in cases of acid reflux and irritable bowel syndrome (IBS).
- **Women's Health**: Acupuncture is employed to manage menstrual irregularities, menopausal symptoms, and infertility.

Evidence

The efficacy of acupuncture has garnered a great deal of academic attention. Although Western medicine still doesn't completely understand how acupuncture works, there is evidence to support its treatment for certain conditions:

Management of Pain: Acupuncture has been shown to alleviate pain, especially headaches and chronic pain, according to many high-quality studies and meta-analyses.

Nausea and Vomiting: Acupuncture, particularly at the P6 acupoint (located on the wrist), help lessen the vomiting and nausea caused by chemotherapy and surgery has been shown.

Mental Health: A more comprehensive understanding of the effects of acupuncture on depression and anxiety is required, but preliminary trials show promise.

For some medical issues, acupuncture has shown promise in randomized controlled studies; the World Health Organization (WHO) has compiled a list of these ailments. To better understand the therapeutic advantages and limits of acupuncture, however, the scientific community is still investigating its processes.

Chiropractic is an alternative medical practice that specializes in the manipulation and adjustment of the spine and other musculoskeletal systems to alleviate pain and other mechanical issues. The basic idea is that when the body's bones, and the spine in particular, are in their correct positions, is essential for optimal health and function.

Origin

Chiropractic care originated in the late 19th century. The founder of chiropractic, it was the first chiropractic adjustment, done in 1895, by Daniel David Palmer. Palmer's theory was that misalignments in the spine, which he termed "subluxations," could interfere with the nervous system and cause a variety of health problems. This concept was revolutionary at the time and laid the foundation for the chiropractic profession.

Theory

The core theory behind chiropractic care is the power to mend itself inherent to every living thing. But this self-repairing mechanism can be impeded by subluxations, which are misalignments or abnormal movements in the joints, particularly those of the spine. These subluxations can lead to pressure on nerves, reduced range of motion, and inflammation, potentially causing pain and dysfunction.

Chiropractors believe that by correcting these subluxations through manual adjustments, they can restore proper nerve function, improve joint mobility, and alleviate pain. This approach highlights the role of the skeleton in general health and wellness.

Practice

Chiropractic treatment primarily involves manual adjustments, also known as spinal manipulative therapy (SMT). These adjustments are designed to realign the spine and other joints, reduce pressure on nerves, and improve overall biomechanics. Chiropractors use a variety of techniques to perform these adjustments, including:

High-Velocity, Low-Amplitude (HVLA) Thrusts: These are the classic chiropractic adjustments that involve a short, quick thrust to realign the joints.

Mobilization: Gentler techniques that stretch the muscles and allow the joints to move in different ways.

Instrument-Assisted Adjustments: Some chiropractors use hand-held instruments to apply controlled force to the spine.

Chiropractic care also often includes patient education on posture, ergonomics, and exercises to prevent future subluxations and maintain spinal health.

Applications

Chiropractic care and a host of other musculoskeletal issues, such as:

A lot of individuals go to chiropractors in hopes of getting some relief from back discomfort.

Neck Pain: Chiropractic adjustments can help alleviate neck pain and associated headaches.

Headaches: Many people find relief from tension headaches and migraines through chiropractic treatment.

Sciatica: Adjustments can help relieve pressure on the sciatic nerve, reducing pain and discomfort.

Chiropractic care is also used for other conditions such as carpal tunnel syndrome, fibromyalgia, and sports injuries.

Evidence

The effectiveness of chiropractic care has been researched extensively. There is evidence to back up its use for certain musculoskeletal conditions, particularly back pain:

Back Pain: Several clinical guidelines and systematic reviews have found chiropractic care to be as effective as other treatments, such as physical therapy and exercise, for acute and chronic back pain.

Neck Pain: Chiropractic adjustments are often recommended as a treatment option for neck pain, with evidence suggesting they can provide relief.

Headaches: Some studies have shown that Low back pain, sometimes known as tension headaches or migraines, may be alleviated with chiropractic treatment.

However, the evidence for chiropractic care's effectiveness in treating other conditions is less clear. While many patients report advantages; more study is required to determine its limits and its uses.

Safety and Considerations

The majority of people feel comfortable with chiropractic therapy as long as it is administered by a qualified specialist. The dangers associated with this therapy are the same as those of any medical procedure, including:

Stroke: Rare but serious complications can include arterial dissection leading to stroke, particularly when the neck is manipulated.

Spinal Injuries: Overly forceful or inappropriate adjustments can cause injuries to the spine.

Patients should discuss the potential benefits and risks with their chiropractor and consider seeking a second opinion if necessary.

Make sure the chiropractor has a valid licensure and a solid grasp of of the patient's medical history to provide appropriate care.

Phytotherapy, botanical medicine, or herbal medicine is only one of the many names for the same ancient practice that has been practiced for thousands of years by people from all walks of life. Herbal medicine is the practice of enhancing and treating health through the use of herbs and plant extracts.

Origin

Herbal medicine has been an integral part of medical practices in cultures around the world, including Western herbalism, Traditional Chinese Medicine (TCM), and the Indian system of medicine known as Ayurveda. Each of these traditions has its own unique approach to herbal medicine, with a vast array of plants used for therapeutic purposes.

Ayurveda: Herbs are used in this traditional Indian medical approach to harmonize the three doshas, or energy centers, in the body: Vata, Pitta, and Kapha and promote health.

Traditional Chinese Medicine (TCM): TCM incorporates herbal medicine as one of its main modalities, often using complex formulas that combine multiple herbs to address health issues.

Western Herbalism: This tradition includes the use of herbs in European and North American cultures, with a focus on the individual properties of plants and their effects on the body.

Theory

The theoretical foundation of herbal medicine is based on the belief that plants contain natural compounds that can help the body heal and maintain health. These compounds can have various biological effects, including those that modulate the immune system, reduce inflammation, and fight against microbes.

Herbal medicine practitioners use their knowledge of plant properties to select appropriate herbs for specific health conditions. They consider factors such as the plant's energetics (warm or cool, moist or dry), its affinity for certain organs or systems, and its overall therapeutic action.

Practice

Herbal remedies can be prepared in numerous forms, each with its own method of administration and therapeutic action:

Teas (Infusions or Decoctions): These are made by steeping herbs in hot water and are often used for their gentle and soothing effects.

Tinctures: Concentrated liquid extracts made by soaking herbs in alcohol or glycerin, allowing for the extraction of active compounds.

Capsules and Tablets: Dried herbs or concentrated extracts are encapsulated for easy dosing and to mask unpleasant tastes.

Topical Applications: These include salves, creams, with skin-applied oils that provide targeted benefits.

Suppositories and Enemas: For conditions where local action in the intestines or other body cavities is desired.

Applications

From minor injuries to long-term illnesses, herbal therapy has a broad variety of applications diseases. Some of the most common applications include:

Common Cold and Flu: Supporting the immune system is a common usage for echinacea and elderberry.

Digestive Issues: Ginger and peppermint can help with nausea and indigestion.

Pain Relief: Turmeric and willow bark are anti-inflammatory and pain relievers.

Sleep Disorders: Valerian and chamomile help people unwind and have a better night's rest.

Cardiovascular Health: Hawthorn and garlic are known for their heart-protective effects.

Hormonal Balance: Herbs like chasteberry and black cohosh are used to support reproductive health.

Evidence

The efficacy of herbal medicine varies widely among different herbs and conditions. Some herbs have been backed by scientific data and have undergone thorough investigation, while others have not.

For instance, ginkgo biloba may enhance cognitive performance, while St. John's Wort may have antidepressant benefits; both herbs have been the subject of extensive scientific study.

Limited Evidence: Many herbs have been used traditionally for centuries but have not been subjected to modern clinical trials. This lack of evidence does not necessarily mean they are ineffective, but it does mean that their safety and efficacy are not fully established.

Safety and Considerations

While herbal medicine is often perceived as natural and therefore safe, it is important to remember that herbs can have potent effects and may interact with other medications. It is crucial It is recommended that those with preexisting health concerns or who are taking other drugs speak with a healthcare provider before beginning any new herbal therapy.

Samuel Hahnemann, a German physician, created homeopathy in the late 18th century as an alternative medical approach. Its foundation rests on an original idea and has its own distinct practices, applications, and evidence base.

Origin

Samuel Hahnemann established homeopathy in the latter part of the 18th century. Dr. Hahnemann was a medical doctor who became disillusioned with the harsh and often ineffective treatments of his time. He developed homeopathy as a more gentle and natural approach to healing.

Theory

The core principle of homeopathy is "like cures like," it is the rule of similar. Based on this idea, it is possible to cure comparable symptoms in a sick person by administering a greatly diluted version of a chemical that produces them in a healthy person.

For example, if a substance causes a healthy person to experience a homeopathic treatment for symptoms such as runny nose and conjunctivitis, that substance might be used to treat someone with allergies or a cold.

Practice

Serial dilution and succussion (vigorous shaking) are the steps used in the potentization process to make homeopathic medications. Water is used to dilute the original material or alcohol and then succussed, which is believed to activate the remedy. This process is repeated multiple times, resulting in extremely high dilutions.

These dilutions often exceed Given Avogadro's number (6.022×10^{23}), it is very improbable that the final solution will include even a trace amount of the initial material. But homeopaths hold the belief that the drug's essence or energy is imprinted on the alcohol or water throughout the dilution procedure, so the alcohol or water remembers the substance and its therapeutic properties properties.

Applications

Whether it's a short-term ailment like the common cold or a long-term problem like arthritis or asthma, homoeopathy may help.

All aspects of a patient's mental, emotional, and physical health are considered when homoeopaths choose a treatment plan.

Evidence

The scientific community generally regards homeopathy as pseudoscience. The main criticism of homeopathy is that, except from the placebo effect, no solid data exists to back up its effectiveness. It has been determined via several meta-analyses and systematic reviews that homeopathic medicines do not work more effective than placebos for treating various conditions.

The high dilutions used in homeopathy mean that the remedies often contain no detectable amount of the active ingredient, which contradicts the fundamental principles of pharmacology and chemistry. This has led to skepticism about the plausibility of homeopathic treatments.

Controversy

The controversy surrounding homeopathy centers due to the lack of strong evidence and an explanation that makes sense from a scientific perspective, supporting its efficacy. Critics argue that the principles of homeopathy, particularly the idea that water can retain a memory of substances it has been in contact with, are not supported by current scientific understanding.

Massage therapy

Massage therapy is an approach of manual therapy that focuses on the soft tissues, such as fascia, tendons, ligaments, and muscles, in order to promote relaxation and overall health. This ancient art form has been around for a very long time and is being used now by many different civilizations all around the globe.

Origin

Massage has been used for therapeutic purposes for millennia. Evidence of massage practices can turn up in the artifacts of long-gone cultures like the Greeks, Egyptians, and Chinese. The Chinese medical texts, such as the Huangdi Neijing, mention massage techniques, while Indian Ayurvedic medicine also includes massage as a key component of treatment. In ancient Egypt, massage was a common medicinal herb in Greece, and, Hippocrates, the father of medicine, recommended massage for joint injuries and other conditions.

Theory

Theoretically, massage therapy is based on the idea of manipulating soft tissues to increase blood flow, calm muscles, and alleviate stress. Massage is believed to have several physiological effects, including:

- **Relaxation Response**: Massage can trigger reduces stress and promotes a feeling of well-being via the body's relaxation reaction.
- **Improved Circulation**: By manipulating the muscles and soft tissues, massage can enhance blood and lymphatic circulation that aids in transporting oxygen and nutrients to cells while also removing metabolic waste.
- **Pain Relief**: Reduced muscular tension and enhanced blood flow are two ways in which massage can ease pain the flow of blood and lymph.

- **Enhanced Immune Function**: Research suggests that massage could improve immunity by stimulating the production of certain immune cells.
- **Practice**

There are numerous types of massage, each with its own techniques and applications:

- **Swedish massage**: Among Westerners, this is the massage style most often used. On the deeper levels of muscle tissue, it makes use of friction methods, lengthy strokes, and kneading.

One method is the application of pressure to the deeper layers of muscle using a deep tissue massage treat chronic muscle tension and pain.

- **Sports Massage**: Designed for athletes, this type of massage helps in order to get ready for a large event, recuperate from it, or perform effectively during training.

By applying pressure to certain locations on the feet, hands, or ears, a practice known as reflexology is practiced. These points are thought to relate to various regions of the body. A key principle of reflexology is that these points can be manipulated to promote health and well-being.

- **Trigger Point Therapy**: The method relies on targeting certain muscle areas that are tender and cause pain when pressed.
- **Applications**

Massage therapy is commonly used for a variety of purposes, including:

- **Stress Relief**: Massage can help reduce alleviate tension and encourage rest, which is good for one's psychological and emotional health.
- **Muscle Tension and Pain**: Massage is effective in relieving muscle tension and pain, making it a popular option for aches and pains include headaches, neck pain, and back trouble.
- **Improved Circulation**: Massage helps alleviate edema and boost lymphatic and blood circulation, which in turn improves the operation of the circulatory system.
- **Injury Rehabilitation**: Massage can be part of a rehabilitation program for injuries, helping to reduce pain and improve mobility.
- **Enhanced Performance**: Athletes often use massage to improve their performance and to recover more quickly from training and competition.
- **Evidence**
- Massage treatment may be helpful for various ailments, according to the available research. To illustrate:
- **Stress and Anxiety**: Massage has been found in several studies to have a calming effect and anxiety by lowering cortisol levels and promoting relaxation.
- **Musculoskeletal Conditions**: Conditions like persistent back pain have shown that massage may alleviate pain and improve function, neck pain, and fibromyalgia.
- **Circulation**: Massage can improve circulation; this is good for your health in general and may aid with the treatment of conditions like edema.

However, the evidence for massage therapy's effectiveness varies, to completely grasp its possible advantages and disadvantages, further study is required.

Naturopathy

The inherent healing potential of the human body is the central tenet of naturopathy, a holistic medical practice. The idea originated in the 19th century and has since evolved into a comprehensive approach to health and wellness that incorporates a variety of natural treatments and therapies.

Origin

Naturopathy emerged in the 19th century as a response to the often harsh and ineffective medical treatments of the time. Early naturopaths believed in nature's restorative powers and the body's recuperative capacities, when provided with the proper nutrients and care. As an alternative medical technique, "naturopathy" gained traction in the late 19th century, when the word was first used.

Theory

The core theory of naturopathy is that the body has an innate the capacity to heal, often called vis medicatrix naturae. Naturopathic practitioners work to support and facilitate this natural healing process through the use of natural therapies and treatments. They focus on identifying and removing obstacles to healing, such as poor diet, environmental toxins, and lifestyle factors, while also supplying the body with healing-supporting nutrients.

Practice

Naturopathic treatments are diverse and can include a variety of modalities, such as:

- **Herbal Medicine**: Herbal medicine is the practice of enhancing health through the use of medicinal herbs and their preparations. Herbal medicines may be prescribed by naturopaths to address specific health conditions.
- **Dietary Changes**: Naturopaths often recommend dietary modifications to support healing and improve overall health. This may include the elimination of certain foods, the addition of nutrient-dense foods, and the use of dietary supplements.
- **Lifestyle Counseling**: Advice on lifestyle factors that can impact health, such as stress management, exercise, sleep hygiene, and avoidance of harmful habits like smoking and excessive alcohol consumption.
- **Physical Therapies**: Treatments such as massage, acupuncture, and hydrotherapy may be used to promote relaxation, reduce pain, and improve physical function.
- **Homeopathy**: Some naturopaths are also trained in homeopathy and may use homeopathic remedies as part of their treatment plan.

Applications

From short-term ailments like the flu to long-term issues like diabetes and heart disease, naturopathy may help. You may use it for preventive care and to promote overall wellness. Naturopathic practitioners often work with people to treat the root causes of their illness instead than only its symptoms.

Evidence

The effectiveness of naturopathic treatments varies widely depending on the specific therapy and the condition being treated. Some naturopathic treatments, such as certain herbal remedies and dietary changes, have strong evidence base and are widely accepted as effective. Others, like homeopathy, are more controversial and lack robust scientific support.

Research into naturopathy is ongoing, to completely comprehend the advantages and disadvantages of different naturopathic therapies, further research is required. It should be mentioned that while the majority of naturopathic treatments are thought to be safe, there are a few that might have negative interactions with conventional medicine or even cause adverse effects. Thus, people should always check with their doctors before beginning a new therapy, particularly if they are already sick or receiving medicine.

Reiki

Reiki is a Japanese energy healing technique that has been used since the late 1800s. The fundamental idea is that all living things are connected by an energy field that is essential for health and well-being.

Origin

Reiki was developed by Mikao Usui, a Japanese Buddhist, in the late 19th century. According to tradition, Usui experienced a spiritual awakening on Mount Kurama, where he received the knowledge of Reiki. He then began to practice and teach this healing method, which quickly gained popularity in Japan and then to other regions of the globe.

Theory

The theoretical foundation of Reiki is the belief in a universal life force energy, known as "Rei," which is the source of all life. This energy is thought to flow through the body and can become blocked or depleted, leading to illness and stress. The body's ability to experience joy and health is enhanced when the life force energy is abundant and unrestricted.

By connecting with the patient's energy field, Reiki practitioners hope to speed up the healing process and alleviate symptoms. Balance. They believe that by transferring energy through their kinesthetic abilities, they are able to alleviate energy blockages and bring the body's energy flow back to its normal state.

Practice

During a Reiki session, the patient remains completely dressed while they lie down on a massage table. It is thought that different locations of the practitioner's hands on or near the recipient's body correlate to different energy centers or chakras. The practitioner may also use light touch or hover their hands slightly above the body.

The practice of Reiki is gentle and non-invasive. The recipient may feel warmth, tingling, or a sense of relaxation during the session. Sessions can vary in length but typically last about an hour.

Applications

Reiki is primarily used for stress reduction and relaxation. It is believed to promote emotional and physical healing by bringing harmony back to the energy systems of the body. The practice of Reiki often used to complement other therapies is appropriate for individuals of any age, and health conditions.

Evidence

The evidence for Reiki's effectiveness is largely anecdotal. Many people report feeling more relaxed and experiencing a sense of well-being after Reiki sessions. However, scientific studies on Reiki have yielded mixed results, more investigation is required to support its assertions.

Reiki has shown promise in a number of research, and it may even have effects on stress reduction, anxiety, and pain management. For example, Reiki has been used in hospital settings to help cancer patients manage pain and reduce anxiety. However, these studies often have limitations, such as finding conclusive results is hindered by limited sample numbers and the absence of control groups.

REFERENCES:

- Reference: U.S. Environmental Protection Agency (EPA). (n.d.). *Catalytic Converters and Emission Control Systems*. [Link](https://www.epa.gov/catalytic-converters-and-emission-control-systems)
- Reference:
  Johnson, T. V. (2009). *Vehicle Emissions and Emissions Control: Past, Present, and Future*. SAE International Journal of Engines, 2(1), 123-138. [Link](https://doi.org/10.4271/2009-01-0189)
- Reference: U.S. Environmental Protection Agency (EPA). (n.d.). *Air Pollution Control Techniques for Industrial Waste*. [Link](https://www.epa.gov/air-pollution-control-techniques-industrial-waste)
- Reference: Cooper, C. D., & Alley, F. C. (2011). *Air Pollution Control: A Design Approach*. Waveland Press.
- Reference: European Environment Agency. (2019). *Air Quality in Europe — 2019 Report*. [Link](https://www.eea.europa.eu/publications/air-quality-in-europe-2019)
- Reference: World Health Organization (WHO). (2021). *Air Pollution*. [Link](https://www.who.int/news-room/fact-sheets/detail/ambient-(outdoor)-air-quality-and-health)

References:

- Reference: Metcalf & Eddy, Inc. (2014). *Wastewater Engineering: Treatment and Resource Recovery*. McGraw-Hill Education.
- Reference: U.S. Environmental Protection Agency (EPA). (n.d.). *Advanced Wastewater Treatment*. [Link](https://www.epa.gov/advanced-wastewater-treatment)
- Reference: U.S. Department of Agriculture (USDA). (n.d.). *Agricultural Runoff and Water Quality*. [Link](https://www.usda.gov/topics/environment/agricultural-runoff-and-water-quality)
- Reference: National Research Council. (2002). *Water Quality and Agriculture*. National Academies Press. [Link](https://doi.org/10.17226/10298)
- Reference: National Oceanic and Atmospheric Administration (NOAA). (n.d.).
  Oil Spills. [Link](https://response.restoration.noaa.gov/oil-and-chemical-spills)
  Fingas, M. (2011). *Oil Spill Science and Technology*. Gulf Professional Publishing.
- Reference: United States Environmental Protection Agency (EPA). (n.d.). *Soil and Groundwater Remediation*. [Link](https://www.epa.gov/superfund/soil-and-groundwater-remediation)
- Reference: EPA. (2017). *Introduction to Phytoremediation*. [Link](https://www.epa.gov/sites/production/files/2015-09/documents/phytoremediation.pdf)
- Reference: U.S. Environmental Protection Agency (EPA). (n.d.). *Pesticides*. [Link](https://www.epa.gov/pesticides)

References:

- Reference: Pimentel, D., & Burgess, M. (2013). Soil Erosion Threatens Food Production. Agriculture, 3(3), 443-463. [Link](https://doi.org/10.3390/agriculture3030443)
- Reference: World Health Organization (WHO). (2018). Environmental Noise Guidelines for the European Region. [Link](https://www.who.int/europe/publications/i/item/9789289053563)
- Reference: European Environment Agency. (2020). Noise in Europe—2020. [Link](https://www.eea.europa.eu/publications/noise-in-europe-2020)
- Reference: U.S. Department of Transportation (DOT). (n.d.). Noise and Transportation. [Link](https://www.transportation.gov/policy/aviation/noise-and-emissions)
- Reference: European Commission. (n.d.). *Noise from Transport*. [Link](https://ec.europa.eu/environment/noise/transport.htm)
- Reference: J. K. Davis et al., "Economic Incentives for Milk Adulteration: A Global Perspective," Journal of Dairy Science, 2019.
- Reference: M. A. Johnson et al., "Impact of Adulteration on the Volume and Sales of Fruit Juices," Journal of Food Engineering, 2020.
- Reference: L. G. Garcia et al., "Adulteration of Olive Oil with Vegetable Oils: Detection and Quantification by Gas Chromatography," Journal of Agricultural and Food Chemistry, 2021.
- Reference: R. K. Patel et al., "Impact of Calcium Carbide on the Shelf Life of Fruits," International Journal of Food Sciences and Nutrition, 2022.

References:

- Reference: S. A. Khan et al., "Artificial Ripening of Fruits with Calcium Carbide: Health Risks and Regulatory Perspectives," Journal of Agricultural and Food Chemistry, 2021.
- Reference: S. B. Lee et al., "Detection of Olive Oil Adulteration Using Near-Infrared Spectroscopy and Chemometrics," Journal of Food Composition and Analysis, 2021.
- Reference: J. K. Davis et al., "Economic Incentives for Milk Adulteration: A Global Perspective," Journal of Dairy Science, 2019.
- Reference: R. G. Patel et al., "Contamination of Food Products with Industrial Waste: Health Risks and Regulatory Implications," International Journal of Food Sciences and Nutrition, 2022.
- Reference: M. A. Smith et al., "Health Risks Associated with Artificial Food Coloring," Journal of Food Science, 2020.
- National Center for Biotechnology Information (NCBI). (n.d.). PubChem Compound Summary for CID 7190, Butylated Hydroxyanisole. Retrieved from https://pubchem.ncbi.nlm.nih.gov/compound/Butylated-Hydroxyanisole
- U.S. Food and Drug Administration (FDA). (2020). Food Additives & Ingredients - Butylated Hydroxyanisole (BHA) and Butylated Hydroxytoluene (BHT). Retrieved from https://www.fda.gov/food/food-additives-ingredients/butylated-hydroxyanisole-bha-and-butylated-hydroxytoluene-bht
- Center for Science in the Public Interest (CSPI). (2010). Food Dyes: A Rainbow of Risks. Retrieved from https://cspinet.org/new/pdf/foodsafety/dyes_factsheet.pdf
- U.S. Food and Drug Administration (FDA). (2018). Color Additives & FDA. Retrieved from https://www.fda.gov/food/food-ingredients-packaging/color-additives

References:

- National Institutes of Health (NIH). (2020). Artificial Sweeteners and Cancer. Retrieved from https://www.cancer.gov/about-cancer/causes-prevention/risk/diet/artificial-sweeteners-fact-sheet
- American Heart Association. (2019). Is It OK to Use Artificial Sweeteners in Place of Sugar? Retrieved from https://www.heart.org/en/healthy-living/healthy-eating/eat-smart/sugar/artificial-sweeteners
- Harvard T.H. Chan School of Public Health. (2020). Trans Fats. Retrieved from https://www.hsph.harvard.edu/nutritionsource/trans-fats/
- U.S. Food and Drug Administration (FDA). (2015). FDA Takes Step to Ban Partially Hydrogenated Oils in Food. Retrieved from https://www.fda.gov/news-events/press-announcements/2015/ucm449162.htm
- National Center for Complementary and Integrative Health (NCCIH). (2020). Monosodium Glutamate (MSG). Retrieved from https://www.nccih.nih.gov/health/monosodium-glutamate
- U.S. Food and Drug Administration (FDA). (2018). Questions and Answers on Monosodium Glutamate (MSG). Retrieved from https://www.fda.gov/food/food-ingredients-packaging/questions-and-answers-monosodium-glutamate-msg
- U.S. Food and Drug Administration (FDA). (2018). Food Additives & Ingredients - Flavoring Agents and Extracts. Retrieved from https://www.fda.gov/food/food-additives-ingredients/flavoring-agents-and-extracts
- National Center for Biotechnology Information (NCBI). (n.d.). PubChem Compound Summary for CID 638175,

References:

- Artificial Flavor. Retrieved from https://pubchem.ncbi.nlm.nih.gov/compound/638175
- U.S. Food and Drug Administration (FDA). (2018). Food Additives & Ingredients - Color Additives. Retrieved from https://www.fda.gov/food/food-additives-ingredients/color-additives
- Center for Science in the Public Interest (CSPI). (2010). Chemical Cuisine. Retrieved from https://cspinet.org/reports/chemcuisine.htm
- U.S. Department of Agriculture (USDA). (2020). Canned Fruits. Retrieved from https://www.choosemyplate.gov/fruits-canned
- American Cancer Society. (2020). Sodium and Canned Foods. Retrieved from https://www.cancer.org/healthy/eat-healthy/canned-foods.html
- U.S. Food and Drug Administration (FDA). (2018). Food Additives & Ingredients - Gold. Retrieved from https://www.fda.gov/food/food-additives-ingredients/gold
- National Center for Biotechnology Information (NCBI). (n.d.). PubChem Compound Summary for CID 23984, Gold. Retrieved from https://pubchem.ncbi.nlm.nih.gov/compound/23984
- U.S. Food and Drug Administration (FDA). (2018). Food Additives & Ingredients - Baking Mixes. Retrieved from https://www.fda.gov/food/food-additives-ingredients/baking-mixes
- Center for Science in the Public Interest (CSPI). (2010). Cake Mixes. Retrieved from https://cspinet.org/new/pdf/foodsafety/cake_mixes.pdf
- "Nanoencapsulation of essential oils as a green technique to enhance their antimicrobial properties in food systems: A

References:

review" (2021).Source: Food Control, Volume 121, 2021, 107574.

- Toxicity, monitoring and biodegradation of organophosphate pesticides: a review Publication date: 2019.
  Summary: ... characteristics of organophosphate pesticides, their environmental issues, analytical ... The site of action of various organophosphates on the electron transport chain of the light ...
- Common mechanism of toxicity: a case study of organophosphorus pesticides
  Publication date:1998. Summary: ... these and other issues using the organophosphorus (OP) class ... of action, but do not cause the same critical toxic response. ... , including the fungicide fosetyl-Al, the plant growth regulator ...
- Carbamate Toxicity - StatPearls: This resource from the National Institutes of Health provides detailed information on carbamates, including common agents, toxic exposure, and health effects.
- Carbamate Toxicity - PubMed: An overview of carbamates, discussing their structural and mechanistic similarities to organophosphates.
- Carbamates: Human Exposure and Health Effects (Research Gate): A detailed PDF discussing the toxic effects of carbamates on human health, including interference with reproductive systems and fetal development.
- N-Methyl Carbamate Insecticides (EPA): Information from the U.S. Environmental Protection Agency on the absorption and toxicity of carbamates.

References:

- Carbamate Insecticide - ScienceDirect: This article provides an overview of carbamates as insecticides, including their short half-life and potential for causing acute intoxication.
- References: Environmental Working Group (EWG). (2023). "Teflon Toxins: Are They Lurking in Your Cookware?" Retrieved from https://www.ewg.org/teflon-toxins/
- Referance:U.S. Environmental Protection Agency (EPA). (2023). "Perfluorooctanoic Acid (PFOA) (C8) and Perfluorooctanesulfonic Acid (PFOS)." Retrieved from https://www.epa.gov/pfoa-pfos
- Consumer Reports. (2023). "What You Need to Know About Nonstick Pans." Retrieved from https://www.consumerreports.org/cookware/nonstick-cookware-safety/
- "Aluminum toxicity in patients with chronic renal failure: Enemy within, foe without" by Alfrey, A. C., American Journal of Kidney Diseases, 1990.
- "Aluminum intoxication" by Alfrey, A. C., Annual Review of Medicine, 1986.
- "Aluminum and bone health" by Sjögren, A., Journal of Internal Medicine, 1996.
- "Effect of food composition on the leaching of aluminum from cooking pans" by Versieck, J., et al., Food Additives & Contaminants, 1986.
- General Information and Benefits "The Benefits of Cooking with Clay Pots" by The Spruce Eats (2020) Link This article discusses the health and flavor benefits of cooking with clay pots, including moisture retention and even heat distribution.
- "Cooking with Clay: The Art of Cooking in Earthen Pots" by Saveur Magazine (2018)

References:

Link This article explores the traditional practice of cooking with clay pots and its modern revival, highlighting the unique flavors and textures achieved.

- Precautions and Tips "How to Use and Care for Your Terracotta Cookware" by Food52 (2017)Link This guide provides detailed instructions on seasoning, cooking with, and cleaning terracotta cookware to ensure its longevity and effectiveness.
- "The Complete Guide to Cooking with Clay Pots" by Serious Eats (2019)
  Link This comprehensive guide covers everything from choosing the right clay pot to specific cooking techniques and maintenance tips.
- Environmental Considerations "Sustainable Kitchen: The Eco-Friendly Benefits of Clay Cookware" by EcoWatch (2021)Link This article discusses the environmental benefits of using clay cookware, emphasizing its sustainability and biodegradability.
- "Why You Should Cook with Terracotta: A Sustainable Choice" by TreeHugger (2020)Link TreeHugger highlights the sustainable aspects of terracotta cookware and its lower carbon footprint compared to metal or synthetic alternatives.
- Scientific Studies"Effect of Cooking Methods on Nutritional and Sensory Quality of Foods" by the Journal of Food Science and Technology (2015)LinkThis study compares different cooking methods, including the use of clay pots, and their impact on the nutritional and sensory qualities of food.
- "Clay Pot Cooking: An Ancient Technique for Modern Kitchens" by the Journal of Ethnic Foods (2018)LinkThis article explores the history and modern applications of clay pot cooking, including its health and environmental benefits.S. Environmental Protection Agency (EPA): "Drinking Water Contaminants"

References:

(https://www.epa.gov/ground-water-and-drinking-water/drinking-water-contaminants)
- "Water Treatment and Distribution" (https://www.epa.gov/water-research/water-treatment-and-distribution)
- World Health Organization (WHO): "Water Quality and Health" (https://www.who.int/news-room/fact-sheets/detail/water-quality-and-health)
- "Waterborne Diseases" (https://www.who.int/news-room/fact-sheets/detail/waterborne-diseases)
- "Guidelines for Drinking-water Quality" (https://www.who.int/water_sanitation_health/dwq/gdwq4/en/) Centers for Disease Control and Prevention (CDC): "Emerging Infectious Diseases" (https://www.cdc.gov/eid/index.html)
- "Antibiotic Resistance Threats in the United States" (https://www.cdc.gov/drugresistance/threat-report-2019/index.html)
- **U.S. Environmental Protection Agency (EPA):** "Drinking Water Contaminants" (https://www.epa.gov/ground-water-and-drinking-water/drinking-water-contaminants)
- "Water Treatment and Distribution" (https://www.epa.gov/water-research/water-treatment-and-distribution)
- "Water Quality and Health" (https://www.who.int/news-room/fact-sheets/detail/water-quality-and-health)
- "Waterborne Diseases" (https://www.who.int/news-room/fact-sheets/detail/waterborne-diseases)
- "Guidelines for Drinking-water Quality" (https://www.who.int/water_sanitation_health/dwq/gdwq4/en/)
- Centers for Disease Control and Prevention (CDC): "Emerging Infectious Diseases" (https://www.cdc.gov/eid/index.html)"Antibiotic Resistance Threats in the United States"

References:

(https://www.cdc.gov/drugresistance/threat-report-2019/index.html)
- Beetroot as a functional food with huge health benefits: Antioxidant, antitumor, physical function, and chronic metabolomics activity Liping Chen1 | Yuankang Zhu2 | Zijing Hu3 | Shengjie Wu1 | Chengtao Jin1
- Bitter Gourd: Health Benefits, Nutrition, and Uses Medically Reviewed by Christine Mikstas, RD, LD on August 31, 2022 Written by WebMD Editorial Contributor
- Health Benefits of Okra Medically Reviewed by Poonam Sachdev on September 12, 2022 Written by WebMD Editorial Contributor
- The Health Benefits of Radishes They are packed with vitamins By Michelle Pugle
  Published on May 15, 2023
- What are the Health Benefits of Cluster Beans? May 22, 2024 Written by Team Diabesmart Medically Reviewed Surabhi KS Nutritionist | Diabetes Educator
- Snake Gourd: A Review of its Nutritional and Medicinal Efficacy Atugwu Agatha Ifeoma1*, Nweze Emilia Ifedilichukwu2, Onyia Vincent Nduka1
- Impressive Health Benefits of Snake Gourd By Michael Jessimy / April 28, 2024 Mustard Greens: Nutrition Facts and Health Benefits Medical Author: Nazneen Memon, BHMS, PGDCR Medical Reviewer: Shaziya Allarakha, MD
- Surprising Health Benefits of Coriander by Meenakshi Nagdeve last updated - March 27, 2024 Medically reviewed by Vanessa Voltolina (MS, RD)
- Medicinal Profile, Phytochemistry, and Pharmacological Activities of Murraya koenigii and Its Primary Bioactive

References:

Compounds Authors: Rengasamy Balakrishnan,1 Dhanraj Vijayraja,2 Song-Hee Jo,1 Palanivel Ganesan,3 In Su-Kim,1,* and Dong-Kug Choi1,

- Everything you need to know about green beans Medically reviewed by Natalie Butler, R.D., L.D. Written by Megan Ware, RDN, L.D. on January 19, 2018
- Green Beans Nutrition Can Help You Fight Cancer and Improve Digestion By Rebekah Edwards October 13, 2023
- Health Benefits of Apples Medically Reviewed by Zilpah Sheikh, MD on January 31, 2024 Written by Alyson Powell Key
- Health benefits of bananas By Zoey Larsen | Apr. 15, 2024 Orange Nutrition Benefits Skin, Gut Health & Immunity By Rachael Link, MS, RD January 10, 2024
- Are strawberries good for you? Benefits, nutrition, and more Medically eviewed by Imashi Fernando, MS, RDN, CDCES — Written by Megan Ware, RDN, L.D. — Updated on July 13, 2023
- Cognition: the new frontier for nuts and berries Peter Pribis, Barbara Shukitt-Hale Available 28 May 2014, Version of Record 18 February 2023.
- What are the benefits of blackberries? Medically reviewed by Natalie Olsen, R.D., L.D., ACSM EP-C — Written by Aaron Kandola on June 7, 2018
- Health benefits of raspberries Medically reviewed by Miho Hatanaka, RDN, L.D. — Written by Megan Ware, RDN, L.D. on October 17, 2019
- Grapes and Cardiovascular Disease Mustali M. Dohadwala [1], Joseph A. Vita

References:

- Properties and Therapeutic Application of Bromelain: A Review Rajendra Pavan, Sapna Jain, Shraddha, and Ajay Kumar*
- Here's Why Mangoes Are So Good for You Although high in sugar, they may control blood sugar levels By Lindsey DeSoto, RD, LD Published on June 22, 2023
- Watermelon and l-Citrulline in Cardio-Metabolic Health: Review of the Evidence 2000–2020
- Benefits of Kiwi Fruit: A Superfood for Your Health Christie Borders, MS, CNS Published in Nutrition 9 min read October 30, 2023 Volume 23, article number 81, (2021)
- Is Papaya Good for You? Adam Meyer Published on November 7, 2022
- Health Benefits of Cherries By Andrea Mathis, M.A., RDN, LD Updated on August 17, 2020
- Health Benefits of Pomegranates Medically Reviewed by Jabeen Begum, MD on May 14, 2024 Written by Katie Cameron, Lori M. King, PhD Published: 11 December 2021
- Plum nutrition facts, benefits, and risks Medically reviewed by Kim Rose-Francis RDN, CDCES, LD, Nutrition — Written by Anna Smith Haghighi on March 30, 2021
- Health Benefits of Guava Medically Reviewed by Poonam Sachdev on July 03, 2023 Written by WebMD Editorial Contributor
- Health Benefits of Lemon Medically Reviewed by Jabeen Begum, MD on March 26, 2024 Written by WebMD Editorial Contributor
- Great Reasons to Add Dragon Fruit to Your Diet Written by Makayla Meixner MS, RDN on May 23, 2018

References:

- Nutritional and Health Benefits of Jackfruit (*Artocarpus heterophyllus* Lam.): A Review R. A. S. N. Ranasinghe, S. D. T. Maduwanthi, and R. A. U. J. Marapana
- Impressive Health Benefits of Gooseberries Written by Elise Mandl, BSc, Msc, APD — Updated on July 13, 2023
- Health Benefits of Mulberries Medically Reviewed by Dany Paul Baby, MD on November 24, 2022
- Acai Berry: 6 Proven Benefits, Including Clear Skin and Weight Loss By Jillian Levy, CHHC January 23, 2020
- Durian Fruit: Potent Smell but Incredibly Nutritious Medical Author: Dr. Sruthi M., MBBS
- Surprising Benefits Of Star Fruit (Carambola) Written by Prisha Raote Posted on Nov 2, 2023
- Are Cranberry Pills Good for You? Benefits, Side Effects and Dosage Written by Erica Julson, MS, RDN, CLT — April 18, 2023
- Apricots: Health Benefits, Nutrition, and Uses Medically Reviewed by Kathleen M. Zelman, RD, LD, MPH on August 22, 2022
- Can figs be beneficial to our health? Medically reviewed by Miho Hatanaka, RDN, L.D. — By Jessica Caporuscio, PharmD on December 4, 2019
- The therapeutic properties and applications of Aloe vera: A review Author links open overlay panelAbid Aslam Maan [a,b], Akmal Nazir [a,b,e], Muhammad Kashif Iqbal Khan [a,b], Tahir Ahmad [b], Rabia Zia [c], Misbah Murid [b], Muhammad Abrar [d]
- Ginseng in Traditional Herbal Prescriptions Ho Jae Park,[1,#] Dong Hyun Kim,[2,3] Se Jin Park,[2,3] Jong Min Kim,[2,3] and Jong Hoon Ryu[1,3,*]

References:

- Tiger Milk Mushroom: A Comprehensive Review of Nutritional Composition, Phytochemicals, Health Benefits, and Scientific Advancements with Emphasis on Chemometrics and Multi-Omics Author overlay panelXi Khai Wong , Cesarettin Alasalvar , Wen Jie Ng , Kah Yaw Ee , Ming Quan Lam , Sui Kiat Chang
- Recent advances in monascus pigments produced by Monascus purpureus: Biosynthesis, fermentation, function, and application Pengfei Gong, … Wei Chen,
- Piper betel leaf extract: anticancer benefits and bio-guided fractionation to identify active principles for prostate cancer management
- Rutugandha Paranjpe1,†, Sushma R.Gundala1,†, N.Lakshminarayana1,2, Arpana Sagwal2 , Ghazia Asif3 , Anjali Pandey4 and Ritu Aneja1,*
- How Should You Use Spirulina? What the Research Says By Regina C. Windsor, MPH, RDN August 31, 2024
- Critical review on chemical compositions and health-promoting effects of mushroom Agaricus blazei Murill Author links open overlay panelKaiyuan Huang [a][b], Hesham R. El-Seedi [c][d], Baojun Xu
- The Nutritional and Pharmacological Potential of Medicinal Mushroom "Ganoderma lucidum (Lingzhi or Reishi)"
- A review of Ganoderma lucidum polysaccharides: Health benefit, structure–activity relationship, modification, and nanoparticle encapsulationpanelFang Kou [a][b][1], Yunfei Ge [b][1], Weihao Wang [a][1], Yuxia Mei [c], Longkui Cao [a], Xuetuan Wei [c], Hang Xiao [d], Xian Wu
- Stability of valeriana-type iridoid glycosides from rhizomes of Nardostachys jatamansi and their protection against

References:

H2O2-induced oxidative stress in SH-SY5Y cells Trung Huy Ngo [a], Ajay Uprety [a], Manju Ojha [a], Yun-Seo Kil [a], Hyukjae Choi [a,b], Soo Young Kim [a], Joo-Won Nam

- Science-Based Benefits of Omega-3 Fatty Acids by Freydis Hjalmarsdottir, MS — Updated on January 17, 2023
- Garcinia Cambogia: Potential Health Benefits vs. Risks By Brittany Lubeck, MS, RDN August 25, 2024
- *Mycobacterium abscessus* disease in lung transplant recipients: Diagnosis and management
  Satish Chandrashekaran,[a] Patricio Escalante,[b,d] and Cassie C. Kennedy[c,e,*]
- Association of Lifelong Intake of Barley Diet with Healthy Aging: Changes in Physical and Cognitive Functions and Intestinal Microbiome in Senescence-Accelerated Mouse-Prone 8 (SAMP8)Chikako Shimizu,[1,*] Yoshihisa Wakita,[1] Makoto Kihara,[2] Naoyuki Kobayashi,[1] Youichi Tsuchiya,[1] and Toshitaka Nabeshima[3,4]
- A review of the effects of mushrooms on mood and neurocognitive health across the lifespanSara Cha [a], Lynne Bell[a], Barbara Shukitt-Hale[b], Claire M. Williams Anti-Inflammatory and Antioxidant Properties of *Piper* Species: A Perspective from Screening to Molecular MechanismsSarvesh Kumar,[1,2] Shashwat Malhotra,[3] Ashok K. Prasad,[3] Erik V. Van der Eycken,[4] Marc E. Bracke,[5] William G. Stetler-Stevenson,[1] Virinder S. Parmar,[3,4,5,*] and Balaram Ghosh[2,*] 11 Proven and Possible Health Benefits of Ginger By Elizabeth Beasley and Nancy LeBrun May 12, 2022
- What Are the Health Benefits of Green Tea? By Lindsay Curtis June 26, 2024

References:

- Atypical Fibroxanthoma of the Conjunctiva in Xeroderma PigmentosumNabeel Shalabi,[a,d] Anat Galor,[a,b] Sander R. Dubovy,[a,c] Jordan Thompson,[a] J. Antonio Bermudez-Magner,[a] and Carol L. Karp[a,*]
- Whole-molecule disorder of the Schiff base compound 4-chloro-*N*-(4-nitrobenzylidene)aniline: crystal structure and Hirshfeld surface analysis Sundararaman Leela,[a,b,*] Ashokkumar Subashini,[b,c] Philip Reji,[d] Kandasami Ramamurthi,[e]
- Cinnamon extract lowers glucose, insulin and cholesterol in people with elevated serum glucoseRichard Anderson [a], Zhiwei Zhan [b], Rencai Luo [c], Xiuhua Guo [d], Qingqing Guo [d], Jin Zhou [e], Jiang Kong [f], Paul A. Davis [g], Barbara J.
- Stoecker Boswellia for osteoarthritis, Zhiqiang Wang, Ambrish Singh, Graeme Jones, Dawn Aitken, Laura L Laslett, Salman Hussain, Pablo García-Molina, Changhai Ding, and Benny Antony
- Isolated Horizontal Gaze Palsy: Observations and Explanations Renee Ewe,[1] Owen B. White,[2,3,*] and Ailbhe Burke[4]
- Chronic administration of the probiotic kefir improves the endothelial function in spontaneously hypertensive rats Andreia G. F. Friques, Clarisse M. Arpini, Ieda C. Kalil, Agata L. Gava, Marcos A. Leal, Marcella L. Porto, Breno V. Nogueira, Ananda T. Dias, Tadeu U. Andrade, Thiago Melo C. Pereira, Silvana S. Meyrelles, Bianca P. Campagnaro, and Elisardo C. Vasquez
- Isolated large vessel pulmonary vasculitis leading to pulmonary artery aneurysm formation: a case report and literature review
- Nima Moghaddam,[1] Bahar Moghaddam,[1] Natasha Dehghan,[1,2] and Nathan W. Brunner

References:

- Benefits of passionflower for anxiety and insomnia by Adrienne Stinson — July 26, 2023
- Antioxidant Properties and Health Benefits:Article: "Honey: A Potent Antioxidant with Multifaceted Therapeutic Applications"**Journal**: Current Neuropharmacology**Year**: 2018
  Authors: K. N. Balasubramanian, S. S. N. Mohan, et al.**Summary**: This article discusses the antioxidant properties of honey and its therapeutic applications, including wound healing and cough suppression.
- **Wound Healing**:**Article**: "The Healing Potential of Honey in Wound Management"
  Journal: Journal of Wound Care**Year**: 2017**Authors**: M. A. Al-Waili
  Summary: This paper reviews the use of honey in wound management and its effectiveness in promoting healing.
- **Cough Suppression**:**Article**: "Honey for Treatment of Cough in Children"
  Journal: Archives of Pediatrics & Adolescent Medicine**Year**: 2007**Authors**: M. L. Paul, M. Behrman, et al.
  Summary: This study compares the effectiveness of honey and over-the-counter cough syrup in relieving cough symptoms in children.
- **Nutritional Value and Health Benefits**:**Article**: "Bee Pollen: Chemical Composition and Therapeutic Applications"**Journal**: Evidence-Based Complementary and Alternative Medicine**Year**: 2015**Authors**: A. Pasupuleti, S. S. Rao, et al.
- **Heart Health**:**Article**: "Effects of Bee Pollen on Cardiovascular Health"**Journal**: Journal of Agricultural and Food Chemistry**Year**: 2016**Authors**: J. Zhang, Y. Li, et al.

References:

- **Allergy Relief:Article**: "Bee Pollen for Allergic Rhinitis: A Systematic Review and Meta-Analysis"**Journal**: Complementary Therapies in Medicine**Year**: 2019**Authors**: M. Zhang, L. Wang, et al.
- **Immune System Boosting:Article**: "Immunomodulatory Effects of Royal Jelly: A Review"**Journal**: Journal of Functional Foods**Year**: 2017**Authors**: S. H. Kim, M. S. Lee, et al.
- **Cognitive Function:Article**: "Royal Jelly and Cognitive Function: A Review"
  Journal: Journal of Traditional and Complementary Medicine**Year**: 2019**Authors**: Y. Zhang, J. Liu, et al.
- **Inflammation Reduction:Article**: "Anti-Inflammatory Effects of Royal Jelly: A Review"
  Journal: Journal of Inflammation Research**Year**: 2018**Authors**: H. Wang, Y. Zhang, et al.
- **Book**: "The Bee Products: Honey, Pollen, Propolis, Royal Jelly"**Authors**: L. B. de Almeida-Muradian, M. Pamplona, et al.**Publisher**: Springer**Year**: 2018
- https://www.rawfoodexplained.com/digestive-physiology-and-food-combining/protein-starch-combinations.html
- https://www.sciencedirect.com/science/article/abs/pii/S0141813021014872
- https://www.sciencedirect.com/science/article/pii/S2213453022001495
- https://www.livestrong.com/article/164642-fruits-that-cause-bloating-gas/
- https://www.mayoclinic.org/diseases-conditions/gas-and-gas-pains/in-depth/gas-and-gas-pains/art-20044739
  References:
- **Environmental Working Group (EWG):Website**: EWG.org

References:

- **Description**: The EWG is a non-profit organization that provides information on environmental health issues. Their Skin Deep database allows consumers to research the safety of personal care products.
- **National Institutes of Health (NIH):Website**: NIH.gov
  Description: The NIH is a leading research institution that provides information on health and safety issues, including the effects of chemicals on human health.
- **Food and Drug Administration (FDA): Website**: FDA.gov
  Description: The FDA regulates food and consumer products in the United States. Their website provides information on the safety of various chemicals, including BPA and phthalates.
- **Consumer Product Safety Commission (CPSC):**
  Website: CPSC.gov **Description**: The CPSC is responsible for protecting consumers from unreasonable risks of injury or death associated with the use of thousands of types of consumer products.
- **World Health Organization (WHO):Website**: WHO.int
  Description: The WHO provides global health guidelines and information on environmental health hazards, including chemical exposures.
- **American Chemical Society (ACS):Website**: ACS.org
  Description: The ACS is a scientific organization that provides resources and information on chemical safety and environmental issues.
- **Occupational Safety and Health Administration (OSHA):Website**: OSHA.govDescription: OSHA provides guidelines and regulations for workplace safety, including information on hazardous chemicals and safe handling practices.

References:

- **Centers for Disease Control and Prevention (CDC):Website**: CDC.gov **Description**: The CDC offers information on environmental health and the impact of chemical exposures on public health.
- **Greenpeace**: **Website**: Greenpeace.org **Description**: Greenpeace is an environmental organization that campaigns for the elimination of toxic chemicals and promotes safer alternatives.
- **The Organic Trade Association:Website**: Organic Trade Association.org**Description**: This association provides information on organic products and their benefits, including reduced exposure to harmful chemicals.
- **The Forest Stewardship Council (FSC):Website**: FSC.org**Description**: The FSC certifies sustainable forestry practices, ensuring that wood and paper products come from responsibly managed forests.
- **The International Agency for Research on Cancer (IARC):Website**: IARC.who.int
  Description: The IARC is part of the WHO and evaluates the carcinogenic risk of chemicals and other agents.
- **U.S. Department of Agriculture (USDA) - MyPlate**:Website: MyPlate is a visual guide to eating a balanced diet. It shows the five food groups (fruits, vegetables, grains, protein, and dairy) and recommends the proportions of each to include in your meals.
- **World Health Organization (WHO) - Balanced Diet**:Website: WHO Nutrition - Balanced DietThe WHO provides guidelines on a balanced diet, emphasizing the importance of variety, moderation, and portion control.

References:

- **Harvard Health Publishing - What Does a Balanced Diet Look Like?**: Article: Harvard Health - Balanced Diet This article from Harvard Health Publishing discusses the components of a balanced diet and provides practical advice on achieving it.
- **American Heart Association - Healthy Eating**: Website: American Heart Association - Healthy Eating The American Heart Association offers recommendations for healthy eating, including tips on incorporating fruits, vegetables, whole grains, lean proteins, and healthy fats into your diet.
- **Dietary Guidelines for Americans**: Website: Dietary Guidelines for Americans The Dietary Guidelines for Americans, published jointly by the USDA and the U.S. Department of Health and Human Services, provides evidence-based nutrition information and advice for people aged 2 years and older.
- **National Institutes of Health (NIH) - Balanced Eating**: Website: NIH - Balanced Eating
  The NIH offers resources on balanced eating, including tips on how to make healthy food choices and maintain a balanced diet.
- **Academy of Nutrition and Dietetics - Eat Right**: Website: Eat Right The Academy of Nutrition and Dietetics provides information on healthy eating, including tips on how to build a balanced plate and make nutritious food choices

Warm-Up
- **American Heart Association**: Warming Up, Cooling Down
- **American Council on Exercise (ACE)**: The Importance of Warming Up
- **National Academies of Sciences, Engineering, and Medicine**: Hydration for Health

References:

- **Centers for Disease Control and Prevention (CDC)**: Hydration for Athletes
- **American College of Sports Medicine (ACSM)**: Selecting the Right Gear for Your Workout
- **Runner's World**: How to Choose the Right Running Shoes
- **Mayo Clinic**: Exercise and Chronic Disease: Get the Facts
- **American Academy of Orthopaedic Surgeons (AAOS)**: Exercise and Fitness
- **American Council on Exercise (ACE)**: The Importance of Cooling Down
- **Verywell Fit**: Why You Should Cool Down After Exercise
- **Centers for Disease Control and Prevention (CDC)**: Physical Activity Guidelines for Americans
- **World Health Organization (WHO)**: Global Recommendations on Physical Activity for Health
- **American College of Sports Medicine (ACSM)**: Finding a Fitness Professional
- **American Heart Association**: Finding a Certified Exercise Professional
- **Overdose and Toxicity: National Institutes of Health (NIH)**: Provides information on dietary supplements, including recommended dosages and upper limits.Office of Dietary Supplements
- **Institute of Medicine (IOM)**: Sets dietary reference intakes (DRIs) for various nutrients, including upper limits to prevent excessive intake.Dietary Reference Intakes
- **Interactions with Medications:Drugs.com**: Offers a drug interaction checker to help identify potential interactions between supplements and medications.Drug Interaction Checker

- **MedlinePlus**: Provides information on drug interactions and supplements.

3. Allergic Reactions:
- **Food and Drug Administration (FDA)**: Offers guidance on food allergies and how to avoid allergens in supplements.

Food Allergies
- **American Academy of Allergy, Asthma & Immunology (AAAAI)**: Provides information on managing allergies and identifying allergens.
  AAAAI

4. Contamination and Adulteration:
- **NSF International**: Certifies supplements for quality and purity.
  - NSF Certified Supplements
- **U.S. Pharmacopeia (USP)**: Sets standards for supplement quality and purity.
  - USP Verified Supplements
- **ConsumerLab.com**: Independently tests and reviews supplements for quality and purity.
  - ConsumerLab.com

5. False Claims and Misleading Advertising:
- **Federal Trade Commission (FTC)**: Regulates advertising and marketing claims for supplements.
  - FTC Consumer Information on Dietary Supplements
- **National Center for Complementary and Integrative Health (NCCIH)**: Provides evidence-based information on supplements.
  - NCCIH

References:

6. Nutrient Imbalances:

- **American Association for Clinical Chemistry (AACC)**: Offers information on nutrient testing and balancing.
  - AACC
- **Academy of Nutrition and Dietetics**: Provides resources on maintaining a balanced diet and using supplements appropriately.
  - Academy of Nutrition and Dietetics

General References:

- **World Health Organization (WHO)**: Provides global guidelines on nutrition and supplementation.
  - WHO Nutrition
- **Centers for Disease Control and Prevention (CDC)**: Offers information on dietary supplements and health.
  - CDC Dietary Supplements

Acupuncture

- **World Health Organization (WHO)**: The WHO has published guidelines and research on the use of acupuncture for various conditions.
- **National Center for Complementary and Integrative Health (NCCIH)**: The NCCIH provides evidence-based information on acupuncture and its effectiveness.
- **Journal Articles**:
  - Linde, K., Allais, G., Brinkhaus, B., Fei, Y., Mehring, M., & Vertosick, E. A. (2020). Acupuncture for the prevention of episodic migraine. Cochrane Database of Systematic Reviews.
  - Vickers, A. J., Cronin, A. M., Maschino, A. C., Lewith, G., MacPherson, H., Foster, N. E., ... & Sherman, K. J.

(2012). Acupuncture for chronic pain: individual patient data meta-analysis. Archives of Internal Medicine.

Chiropractic Care

➤ **American Chiropractic Association (ACA)**: The ACA provides information on chiropractic care and its applications.

➤ **Journal Articles**:
- Gross, A., Langevin, P., Burnie, S. J., Bedard-Brochu, M. S., Empey, B., Dugas, E., ... & Brønfort, G. (2015). Manipulation and mobilisation for neck pain contrasted against an inactive control or another active treatment. Cochrane Database of Systematic Reviews.
- Rubinstein, S. M., van Middelkoop, M., Assendelft, W. J., de Boer, M. R., & van Tulder, M. W. (2011). Spinal manipulative therapy for chronic low-back pain. Cochrane Database of Systematic Reviews.

Herbal Medicine

➤ **National Center for Complementary and Integrative Health (NCCIH)**: The NCCIH offers resources on herbal medicine and its uses.

➤ **World Health Organization (WHO)**: The WHO provides guidelines on traditional medicine, including herbal remedies.

➤ **Journal Articles**:
- Barnes, J., Anderson, L. A., & Phillipson, J. D. (2007). Herbal medicines. Pharmaceutical Press.
- Ernst, E. (2002). The efficacy of herbal medicine—An overview. Fundamental & Clinical Pharmacology, 16(5), 405-409.

References:

Homeopathy
- National Center for Complementary and Integrative Health (NCCIH): The NCCIH provides information on homeopathy and its evidence base.
- Journal Articles:
  - Shang, A., Huwiler-Müntener, K., Nartey, L., Jüni, P., Dörig, S., Sterne, J. A., ... & Egger, M. (2005). Are the clinical effects of homoeopathy placebo effects? Comparative study of placebo-controlled trials of homoeopathy and allopathy. The Lancet, 366(9487), 726-732.
  - Ernst, E. (2010). Homeopathy: What does the "best" evidence tell us? Medical Journal of Australia, 192(8), 458-460.

Massage Therapy
- American Massage Therapy Association (AMTA): The AMTA provides resources on massage therapy and its benefits.
- Journal Articles:
  - Field, T. (2014). Massage therapy research review. Complementary Therapies in Clinical Practice, 20(4), 224-229.
  - Moyer, C. A., Rounds, J., & Hannum, J. W. (2004). A meta-analysis of massage therapy research. Psychological Bulletin, 130(1), 3-18.

Naturopathy
- **American Association of Naturopathic Physicians (AANP)**: The AANP provides information on naturopathy and its principles.

References:

➤ Journal Articles:
- Sarris, J., & Wardle, J. (2018). Integrative naturopathy for mental health: A systematic review. Journal of Affective Disorders, 235, 165-172.
- Riley, D. S., & Blair, J. (2016). Naturopathy and conventional medicine: A multidisciplinary review of their effectiveness in the treatment of chronic diseases. Advances in Integrative Medicine, 3(1), 1-10.

Reiki
➤ International Center for Reiki Training (ICRT): The ICRT provides resources on Reiki and its practice.
➤ Journal Articles:
- Olson, K., Hanson, J., & Michaud, M. (2012). A phase II trial of Reiki for the management of pain in advanced cancer patients. Journal of Pain and Symptom Management, 44(2), 225-234.
- Wardell, D. W., & Engebretson, J. (2011). Review of explanatory mechanisms for the effectiveness of Reiki therapy. Journal of Alternative and Complementary Medicine, 17(1), 7-12.
- IARC Monographs on the Evaluation of Carcinogenic Risks to Humans, Volume 102 (2011): Non-Ionizing Radiation, Part 2: Radiofrequency Electromagnetic Fields.
- Cardis, E., et al. (2011). "Risk of brain tumours in relation to estimated RF dose from mobile phones: results from five Interphone countries." Occupational and Environmental Medicine.
- Frei, P., et al. (2011). "Use of mobile phones and risk of brain tumours: update of Danish cohort study." BMJ.

References:

- National Toxicology Program (NTP) (2018). "Cell Phone Radio Frequency Radiation Studies."
- Effect of electronic gadgets on the eyes of different age groups Ravindra Kumar Manik[1*], Hiba Khan[2], Anshu Kumar Singh[2] Effects of Electronic Devices on Vision in Students Age Group 18-25 August 2021,Annals of Medical and Health Sciences Research 11(7):1572-157
- Electromagnetic fields and health effects—epidemiologic studies of cancer, diseases of the central nervous system and arrhythmia-related heart disease
- Biological effects from electromagnetic field exposure and public exposure standards publication date:2008.Excessive use of electronic devices among children and adolescents is associated with musculoskeletal symptoms, visual symptoms, psychosocial health, and quality of life: a cross-sectional study.
- The health status of adults on the autism spectrum publication date:2015.
- Electromagnetic fields and health effects—epidemiologic studies of cancer, diseases of the central nervous system and arrhythmia-related heart diseaseClinical characteristics, pathophysiology, and management of noncentral nervous system cancer-related cognitive impairment in adults publication date:2015.
- Longitudinal assessment of late-onset neurologic conditions in survivors of childhood central nervous system tumors: a Childhood Cancer Survivor Study report publication date:2018.
- Wired for threat: clinical features of nervous system dysregulation in 80 children publication date:2018.

References:

- mpact of vision loss among survivors of childhood central nervous system astroglial tumors publication date:2016.
- who receive Cancer Therapy: pathophysiology, course, monitoring, management, prevention, and Research Directions: a scientific statement from the American Heart ... publication date:2013.
- Digital health innovations to improve cardiovascular disease carepublication date:2020.
- Association, European Association of Preventive Cardiology, Association of Cardiovascular Nursing and Allied Professionals, Patient Forum, and the Digital Health ...publication date:2021.The risky chemical lurking in your wallet
- New research finds that the BPA in cash register receipts can be absorbed through skin. Published: March 29, 2014
- Sparkling Water: How Healthy Is Carbonation? By Heather Jones Published on November 05, 2023
- Systematic review: the effects of carbonated beverages on gastro-oesophageal reflux disease T. Johnson, L. Gerson, T. Hershcovici, C. Stave, R. Fass First published: 09 February 2010
- Association between Consumption of Carbonated Beverages and Dental Erosion – A Systematic Review October 2021 Journal of Indian Association of Public Health Dentistry 19(4):240
- "Chemical composition and health benefits of Angelica gigas: A review" by J. Kim et al., Journal of Ethnopharmacology, 2019.
- "Immunomodulatory effects of Angelica gigas polysaccharides on macrophages" by H. Lee et al., International Journal of Biological Macromolecules, 2018.

References:

- "Anti-inflammatory effects of Angelica gigas Nakai extract in lipopolysaccharide-stimulated RAW 264.7 macrophages" by S. Park et al., Journal of Ethnopharmacology, 2017.
- "Antioxidant activity of Angelica gigas Nakai extract and its active components" by Y. Jung et al., Food Chemistry, 2016.
- "Effects of Angelica gigas Nakai on menopausal symptoms and lipid metabolism in postmenopausal women: A double-blind, randomized, placebo-controlled study" by J. Kim et al., Menopause, 2015.
- "Vasodilatory and hypotensive effects of Angelica gigas Nakai extract in spontaneously hypertensive rats" by H. Lee et al., Journal of Cardiovascular Pharmacology, 2014.
- "Traditional uses, phytochemistry, and pharmacology of Angelica gigas Nakai: A review" by S. Lee et al., Journal of Traditional and Complementary Medicine, 2019.
- Health benefits of Ceylon cinnamon (Cinnamomum zeylanicum): a summary of the current evidence P Ranasinghe[1], P Galappaththy
- Medicinal properties of 'true' cinnamon (*Cinnamomum zeylanicum*): a systematic review

Priyanga Ranasinghe,[1] Shehani Pigera,[1] GA Sirimal Premakumara,[2] Priyadarshani Galappaththy,[1] Godwin R Constantine,[3] and Prasad Katulanda[3]

- Cinnamomum zeylanicum: Morphology, Antioxidant Properties and Bioactive Compounds April 2021 DOI:10.5772/intechopen.97492 LicenseCC BY 3.0
- Cinnamomum zeylanicum: Morphology, Antioxidant Properties and Bioactive Compounds April 2021 DOI:10.5772/intechopen.97492

References:

- Cinnamon: A Multifaceted Medicinal Plant Pasupuleti Visweswara Rao 1 , 2 ,* and Siew Hua Gan 2
- Evaluation of pharmacodynamic properties and safety of *Cinnamomum zeylanicum* (Ceylon cinnamon) in healthy adults: a phase I clinical trialPriyanga Ranasinghe,[1] Ranil Jayawardena,[2] Shehani Pigera,[1] Wasundara Sevwandi Wathurapatha,[1] Hasitha Dhananjaya Weeratunga,[3] G. A. Sirimal Premakumara,[3] Prasad Katulanda,[4] Godwin Roger Constantine,[4] and Priyadarshani Galappaththy[1]
- Evidence-Based Health Benefits of Cinnamon Written by Joe Leech, MS — Updated on October 24, 2023
- *Paeonia japonica* root extract protects hepatocytes against oxidative stress through inhibition of AMPK-mediated GSK3β Author links open overlay panelHae Li Ko [a], Eun Hye Jung [a], Dae Hwa Jung [b], Jae Kwang Kim [a], Sae Kwang Ku [a], Young Woo Kim [a], Sang Chan Kim [a], Rongjie Zhao [c], Chul Won Lee [a], Il Je Cho [a]
- Paeonia Health Benefits (White Peony Root) By: Van_Der_Linden August 2018Genus
- *Paeonia*: A comprehensive review on traditional uses, phytochemistry, pharmacological activities, clinical application, and toxicology Author links open overlay panelPei Li [a,b], Jie Shen [a,b], Zhiqiang Wang [c], Shuangshuang Liu [a,b], Qing Liu [a,b], Yue Li , Chunnian He , Peigen Xiao
- The Potential Benefits and Side Effects of the White Peony Rootby Kirsten Nunez on October 2020
- *Paeonia lactiflora* Root Extract and Its Components Reduce Biomarkers of Early Atherosclerosis via Anti-Inflammatory and Antioxidant Effects In Vitro and In VivoMin Jeong Kim,[1]

References:

Hyun-Hee Kang,[2] Yeung Jin Seo,[3] Kyung-Min Kim,[4] Young-Jun Kim,[2,*] and Sung Keun Jung[1,5,]

➢ Exploring the pathways of drug repurposing and *Panax ginseng* treatment mechanisms in chronic heart failure: a disease module analysis perspective. Chengzhi Xie, Ying Zhang, Baochen Zhu, Lin Yang, Jianxun Ren & Na Lang

➢ Beneficial effects of *Panax ginseng* for the treatment and prevention of neurodegenerative diseases: past findings and future directionsKi Hyun Kim,[1,☆] Dahae Lee,[1,☆] Hye Lim Lee,[2] Chang-Eop Kim,[2] Kiwon Jung,[3,*] and Ki Sung Kang[2,*]

➢ Chemical constituents of *Panax ginseng* and *Panax notoginseng* explain why they differ in therapeutic efficacyAuthor links open overlay panelHanbing Liu [a 1], Xiaoyan Lu [b 1], Yang Hu [b], Xiaohui Fan [a b]

➢ Pharmacological potential of ginseng and its major component ginsenosidesZubair Ahmed Ratan,[1] Mohammad Faisal Haidere,[2] Yo Han Hong,[3] Sang Hee Park,[4] Jeong-Oog Lee,[5] Jongsung Lee,[3,4,**] and Jae Youl Cho[3,4]

➢ Milk thistle (Silybum marianum): A concise overview on its chemistry, pharmacological, and nutraceutical uses in liver diseasesLudovico Abenavoli [1], Angelo A Izzo [2], Natasa Milić [3], Carla Cicala [2], Antonello Santini [2], Raffaele Capasso [4]

➢ Science Backed Of Milk Thistle By Emily HulseAll You Need to Know About Milk thistle and How it can Improve Liver Health!By Wellbeing Nutrition on 14 July 2022

➢ *Crataeva nurvala* Bark (Capparidaceae) Extract Modulates Oxidative Stress-Related Gene Expression, Restores Antioxidant Enzymes, and Prevents Oxidative Stress in the Kidney and Heart of 2K1C Rats Ishrat Jahan,[1] Proma Saha,[1] Tammana Tabassum Eysha Chisty,[1] Kaniz Fatima Mitu,[1] Faizul

References:

- Islam Chowdhury,[1] Khondoker Shahin Ahmed,[2,3] Hemayet Hossain,[2] Ferdous Khan,[1] Nusrat Subhan,[1] and Md. Ashraful Alam[1]
- Botanical description, phytochemistry, traditional uses, and pharmacology of Crataeva nurvala Buch. Ham.: an updated review December 2020 Future Journal of Pharmaceutical Sciences
- Flaxseed Bioactive Compounds: Chemical Composition, Functional Properties, Food Applications and Health Benefits-Related Gut MicrobesAbdul Mueed,[1,†] Sahar Shibli,[2,†] Sameh A. Korma,[3,4] Philippe Madjirebaye,[1] Tuba Esatbeyoglu,[5,*] and Zeyuan Deng[1,*]
- Dietary Flaxseed as a Strategy for Improving Human HealthMihir Parikh,[1,2,3] Thane G. Maddaford,[1,2,3] J. Alejandro Austria,[1,2,3] Michel Aliani,[2,4] Thomas Netticadan,[1,2,5] and Grant N. Pierce[1,2,3,]
- Flaxseed and Its Nutritional Benefits By Brittany Lubeck, MS, RDN Published on June 09, 2023Shilajit (Mumie): Current Status of Biochemical, Therapeutic and Clinical Advances Tanuja Mishraa , Harcharan S. Dhaliwala , Karan Singhc and Nasib Singha,b
- Evaluation of the effect of purified aqueous extract of shilajit in modifying cardiovascular risk with special reference to endothelial dysfunction in patients with type 2 diabetes mellitusniranjan k1, ramakanth g.S.H1*, nishat fatima2, usharani p3safety and efficacy of shilajit (mumie, moomiyo) sidney j. Stohs*
- Shilajit: A Natural Phytocomplex with Potential Procognitive Activity Carlos Carrasco-Gallardo, Leonardo Guzman, and Ricardo B. Maccioni

References:

Disclaimer:

"The information provided in this document is intended for educational and informational purposes only. It is not a substitute for professional advice or treatment. Readers are encouraged to consult with qualified health professionals regarding any health concerns or before making any decisions based on the information provided."

www.ingramcontent.com/pod-product-compliance
Lightning Source LLC
LaVergne TN
LVHW091617070526
838199LV00044B/826